cancer
POSITIVE

*The Role of the Mind
in Tackling Cancers*

Dr James Colthurst, MBBS, BSc.,
MFHom., MBA, FRCS (Ed.)

with Patrick Scrivenor

Michael O'Mara Books Limited

First published in Great Britain in 2003 by
Michael O'Mara Books Limited
9 Lion Yard, Tremadoc Road
London SW4 7NQ

A CIP catalogue record for this book
is available from the British Library

ISBN 1-85479-860-X

Designed and typeset by Martin Bristow

www.mombooks.com

Printed and bound in Great Britain
by Cox & Wyman, Reading, Berkshire

Contents

Foreword

Why read this book?

This book is written at the request of patients and other doctors. The shock of a serious diagnosis is considerable and patients will not necessarily be able to take in everything the doctor has to say to them. Both patients and doctors have said that to have something to read after the consultation would be of great help. I hope the book will provide a range of 'tools' and psychological aids to help patients, along with their friends and families, who find themselves confronted by cancer, or indeed any other serious illness.

Over the last ten years I have seen an increasing number of patients with malignancy and other serious illnesses. They were often despondent, confused and, more commonly than not, extremely frightened. Much of their fear arose from feeling powerless. They had no idea that there was anything they could do to help themselves.

Learning how to live – not how to die

This book is about *living*, not dying. It is intended to help four main groups:

1. Those who have a cancer

2. Those at risk of cancers

3. Those who know or are related to someone who has cancer

4. Those who are interested in having a cancer-free life!

Can we improve recovery from cancers?

In spite of advances in our understanding of cancers, recovery rates have not significantly improved – at least not enough! The advent of radiotherapy in the forties and chemotherapy in the fifties and sixties gave doctors two extra weapons. Huge sums have since been invested in research of multitudinous kinds, but the promises of improvement made twenty-five years ago have not been realized. Doctors, who would naturally like to produce encouraging statistics for their patients, often find it difficult to do so. Consequently, they often have little choice except to present outcome and recovery statistics in a discouraging way. This, itself, may have an important impact on the patient.

Powerful though they may be, conventional, hospital-based treatments are not the whole story. The mental and physical approach of the patient – before diagnosis, during treatment and after treatment – is vitally important. And here the layman – patient, friend or relative – can play a crucial (and exciting) part in the process of recovery.

Is the book about 'positive thinking'?

The book is not so much about positive thinking as about targeted or focused thinking.

At this point, perhaps I should say something about

myself, and my reasons for writing *Cancer Positive*. I have had an interest in cancers for twenty years. I am an advocate of a broad approach to the techniques associated with the treatment of and recovery from cancers. These may include surgery, radiotherapy and chemotherapy, but I also recommend, use and teach the less frequently encountered procedures of homeopathy, neurolinguistic programming (NLP) and electro stimulation, amongst others.

I am a medical doctor and a surgeon, as well as a fully qualified practitioner of homeopathic medicine. I have had a growing interest in cancers in recent years and have used the approaches in this book to involve many patients in their own treatments. I have achieved encouraging results in some difficult conditions through emphasis on a broad approach to the illness, including the role of the mind in a patient's condition.

This book seeks to put into practice my many years' experience, explaining some psychology of diseases, identifying the psychological pitfalls to avoid and detailing the advantages of certain psychological exercises and mental attitudes, as well as some practical physical tools.

Above all, I believe in the individual patient, the uniqueness of each patient's condition and needs and the importance of stimulating the patient's attitude and mental approach.

This book sets out to tap the potential of psychological and other approaches to cancers. As well as identifying some pitfalls to avoid, it also explains the advantages of developing certain exercises and of fostering certain mental attitudes: relatively simple ways to improve a tricky situation.

Most of all, its purpose is to persuade patients, their families, friends and doctors to recognize that each patient is unique and to demonstrate how many apparently small things can contribute to a considerable change in outcome.

The simple guidelines in this book include physical as well as mental approaches. These aim to convert what may seem 'awful' into a situation which can even make patients 'thankful'. A serious illness can be used as a warning for the patient to create new approaches to their life. Jung was one of several people who regarded illness as a sign 'that the gods were talking'. Let us have a conversation then!

Introduction

The mental and physical exercises described in this book may seem unexpected from a mainstream medic, let alone a surgeon, but they are the result of a progressive journey in pursuit of everything I can find to help my patients recover. I have included all those approaches that I have found particularly effective and I recommend them because they have worked consistently for the last fifteen years as a supplement to other, more conventional treatment. They are not intended to replace or conflict with other treatment.

Your thoughts really can affect your body – an example

It is a proven and accepted phenomenon that the mind can influence the condition of your body, but many people need evidence to be convinced of this.

There is a simple test – the Lemon-Juice Visualization Test – that can provide evidence in many people. It appears in detail on pages 69–71, but a brief explanation here makes the point.

Imagine yourself to be in a desert. It is very, very hot. You are thirsty and your mouth is dry. You are offered a chilled lemon segment to suck. Allow it to rest on your tongue for a moment; then, slowly, sink your teeth into the lemon segment. Notice how it feels, notice the taste, notice the coolness and notice the sharpness of the lemon segment as the taste spreads around your mouth.

When patients have visualized this thoroughly, I ask them what they feel. The overwhelming majority feel increased saliva in their mouths. I point out that the extra saliva is real – and a significant body response – but a response caused by a complete 'fiction', in the form of their imagination; the lemon segment never existed! They have demonstrated, very powerfully, the power of thought over their own body. A thought process, lasting probably not much over a minute or two, has brought about a change in their body involving considerable harnessing of the central nervous system. It is not a big step to accept that much *smaller* thought processes spread *over a longer time* – such as an extended feeling of stress, fear or depression – could have a much greater impact on some part of their body.

The immune system is known mainly as a defence against disease. One job it does is to 'recognize' abnormal molecules in our body; to package them for processing and to arrange for the immune cells to destroy them. Because millions of cells are replaced in our bodies all the time, errors leading to abnormal protein can occur. The errors are more common in a body challenged by pollutants, foods and sunlight, for example.

An immune system that is working normally will spot the errors and remove the abnormal cells before they cause any trouble. The immune system can be regarded as a series of amplifiers where the output from one process feeds into the next – the immune 'cascade'. A 'quiet' signal (such as a worried thought, for example) at the start of the cascade is amplified to cause massive results at the end. The elaborate, brilliant immune system is also rather delicate.

In such a sensitive system, prolonged mental stress (for example leading to increased output from the adrenal glands) is likely to overload the individual's system as its results accumulate and magnify. If left untreated it might stop the immune system working properly. This might allow abnormal cells to accumulate to dangerous levels.

The study of this phenomenon of the effect of the mind on the immune system has been well described by Jean Borysenko and Miroslav Borysenko in their book *The Power of the Mind to Heal* (Dr Joan Borysenko was a Professor of Cell Biology at the Tufts University School of Medicine). What was originally thought by some to be a weak hypothesis has turned out to be theoretically demonstrable.

If our cellular make-up is determined by our genetic inheritance, creating the raw materials with which our bodies function, so other forces can determine how these raw materials behave. We may not be able to see these hidden forces and we may only just be able to measure some of them, but we can see their results. Some of these forces will be influenced by our conscious and unconscious thoughts. If we look carefully at the time scales of cancers forming (and several other illnesses, too), it is clear that some life events can lead to electrical changes – or 'field-changes' – in the body. This 'field-change' can become like a seed-bed in which cancer cells and other cells can alter and grow. By learning how to accept and control these hidden forces, we may be able to reduce the chance of that disease 'seed-bed' forming. If we correct the field, abnormal cells may not be able to survive.

If a cancer has been fully removed and good treatment given, that *may* be the end of it. However, it is possible that a number of 'recurrences' happen because the electro-magnetic field disturbance has remained, even though the cells have been removed. New cells growing in that electromagnetic seed-bed may become altered in the same way as those they replaced – like trying to grow healthy new seeds in contaminated ground. Removing the stresses and strains that can trigger electromagnetic changes therefore becomes a top priority.

Are you stronger than a blade of grass?

If we drill holes in concrete or tarmac we use drills or jack hammers, exerting huge forces to make often irregular holes. It is not so much the sharpness of the bit that makes the difference but how hard it is. A blade of grass, on the other hand, can push its way through tarmac, and sometimes concrete, and when it emerges *it is still soft and flexible*. Maybe we can tap similar forces to help our bodies repair themselves, and even if we cannot, the 'blade of grass' is a very useful example to follow when we look for our powers of recovery!

You are in charge – and capable of it!

And that is the primary theme of this book. Your fate is in your hands. There is an enormous amount *you* can do to improve your outcome. This book will not only make that clear to you, but also equip you with the necessary practical and psychological tools for success.

Is this book about dying? As mentioned earlier – emphatically not! It is about living – about the important part your way of life plays both in illness and in recovery. On one occasion at the Bristol Cancer Help Centre an angry lady from a group of patients (who turned out to be a doctor!) asked at the end of the first day why I had not mentioned dying yet. I told her that I was increasingly unclear when 'death' happened. Of course, physiologically it may be defined by the end of brain or heart activity. However, in disease maybe there is an earlier 'death' when the spirit of the individual is diminished and 'dis-ease' enters a weakened system? For some, this weakness arises when they suffer a shock; for others, redundancy; for others a badly suited job.

On that occasion at Bristol I mentioned certain jobs and professions which I thought suppressed the spirit! I believe that a huge contribution can be made to avoiding and recovering from disease if the *spirit* is restored.

That is why, throughout this book, I emphasize that the *whole* of your life influences your health. It is in the art of living healthily – in its widest sense – that the best chances of recovery lie.

Many things in this book have already benefited patients and they tell me that is why, spirits restored, they asked me to write it.

The tools described in this book have come from all sorts of places and the origins of some may be lost in the mists of time. I am particularly grateful for suggestions made by many encouraging professionals. These include Anthony Robbins (known for *Awaken the Giant Within* and *Unlimited Power*), The Living Game seminar, and some of the team at the Bristol Cancer Help Centre. There are many others who have contributed to the challenging world of cancer treatment and I hope that readers will realize that this book may be merely a beginning for them, rather like a framework to build on. *If only one of the approaches in this book* succeeds in improving the course of someone's journey through cancer or another serious illness, then it has been worthwhile writing it!

Ralph Waldo Trine wrote in his book *In Tune With the Infinite* that 'the time will come when the work of the physician will not be to treat and attempt to heal the body, but to heal the mind, which in turn will heal the body'. That book was first published in 1899. The only addition I would make – over one hundred years later – is that the physician might now consider teaching the *patient* how to use their mind to heal their body.

The format of the book:

- Reducing the causes of cancers
- Understanding what you can do
- Creating a target to aim for
- Making it happen
- Keeping up the progress

Chapter 1
Reducing the Causes
– Stop the rot!

Making it harder for cancers to form or stay in us

The role of genetics

There seems to be a genetic predisposition to certain cancers, and this fact tends to encourage a fatalistic attitude among those who feel at risk. But it is very far from the case that everyone with a genetic tendency in the family will contract a cancer. Consider a stick as an example: Genes have determined its structure – with weak points and strong points. If the stick is put under a strain it will break somewhere. The *site* of breakage may be determined by the genetic code, but the *strain* is an external force. If two sticks are different, the same load will break them in different places. There may not be anything we can do to alter our genetic structure, but there is a considerable amount we can do to alter the strain on it.

Stress – physical and mental

In general terms we are all at risk of cancers – just as we are at risk of many other serious illnesses. The causes of cancers are complex and not yet wholly understood, but there are major 'areas of risk' that we can home in on to improve our understanding of our exposure to risk.

'Stresses' which may help cancers to form:

- Environmental toxins – pesticides, foods, cleaners etc

- Physical agents – sunlight, magnetic fields

- Mental stress – bereavement, work, home, relationships.

Environmental toxins

Samuel Epstein, Professor of Environmental Medicine at the University of Illinois, stated as early as 1997 that by 2003 nearly 50 per cent of people living in the western world would experience cancer at some stage in their lives. This statistic has changed from the 1920s, when it was around 1-in-5, through 1-in-3 twenty years ago, to about 1-in-2.5 now. We will approach the '1-in-2' mark more or less at the time this book is published.

There are many reasons for this increase. Among them are environmental toxins, *including those found around the home*. Some heavily promoted household cleaning products and weedkillers, for example, are significantly toxic.

Farmers are often strongly criticized for indiscriminate spraying of herbicides and insecticides. Crop spraying in developed countries, however, is usually carefully controlled. These sprays are, by and large, delivered by people who are experienced, even trained, in delivering them. Contrast this to garden weedkillers. Frequently they are applied in a container whose measurements may not be clear. The user will often add a 'little bit more' for good measure – if it's five parts to the container, they'll use ten just to make *really* sure the weeds are killed! Many weedkillers are used in summer, when people are wearing less clothing, with bare feet. Children, with their vulnerable systems, are even closer to sprayed ground. Most domestic gardeners don't apply weedkillers very often. They are not experienced and they wear next to no protective clothing, often walking over the spray that they have just delivered.

It is vitally important to read the instructions and take adequate precautions, like wearing protective clothing. Just because a weedkiller is on open sale does not mean it is safe to splash around.

Is your kitchen a hidden-hazard zone?

Inside the house things may be even worse. Heavy advertising convinces people that 'dangerous bacteria' lurk everywhere – especially in the kitchen and the bathroom – and an enormous quantity of chemical disinfectant is sold to combat this 'threat'. However, spraying kitchen surfaces and disinfecting every lavatory bowl in the house does not kill all the bugs. Over-disinfecting may also be generating 'hidden' toxicity by an accumulation of chemicals in the house. These may then be absorbed through the skin, inhaled, or eaten (by preparing food on 'chemically-cleaned' surfaces, for example).

Most common bacteria dislike dry conditions, so by wiping surfaces and allowing them to dry most of these bacteria will not grow. Wooden chopping boards have natural antibacterial properties. Dishcloths and drying-up cloths and towels should be put somewhere where they can dry properly after use.

In the rest of the house, many carpets are treated with anti-fungal chemicals, and gases given off by the carpets can be a further source of trouble. In temperate climates many people air their houses less than they used to, either because it's expensive to heat the house or for security reasons. So toxins don't have a chance to escape. They can be easily absorbed into the surfaces of the house.

Fortunately, Professor Epstein offers advice on how to avoid household toxins in his book *The Safe Shopper's Bible*. He lists a large number of household products (albeit under American brand names) such as cleaning products, beauty products and weedkillers. He lists the ingredients of these products and explains which ones are harmful and what is dangerous about them. He concludes each section of the book with a list of safe alternative products.

Already, therefore, there is something you can do to reduce your risk of contracting a cancer, or to improve your chances of recovery if you have a cancer. Reduce your toxic intake. By reducing the toxicity around you, you can lessen the demands on your immune system and allow the body to focus on recovery. For example, there is no point in a patient with lung cancer having treatment while continuing to smoke. The danger of household products is not as obvious a danger as smoking, but it is real none the less. By choosing safe products, patients are already helping themselves – at the very least by reducing the load on the immune system.

Foods: Pesticides, food preservatives, colourants and flavours are used in many foods. To these must be added the growth promoters and antibiotics which seem to have become the staple intake of many animals. The easiest way to reduce your intake of food pollutants is to eat organic – or as nearly as you can.

Water: Tap water may not be all that safe, either! The chemicals that we excrete or that are put down the sink may well find their way in to our drinking water. Groundwater may be contaminated from landfill sites. The contraceptive pill has now led to higher oestrogen levels in tap water. These hormones may be responsible for increases in hormone-based tumours. You can avoid water-borne toxins by filtering or processing the water. Charcoal filters will remove a great deal of trouble but the gold standard of processing is probably a reverse-osmosis filter system. Ordinary tap water can still be used for washing, bathing and washing the dishes.

Smoking – increasing the risks

One of the most commonly used toxins contributing to cancers is cigarette smoking. Commonly associated with lung cancer, it is likely that it raises the occurrence of cancers of many kinds throughout the body. For example, the tar that builds in lungs moves up to the throat at night when the paralyzing effect of smoking on the cleaning mechanism has worn off. The tar-containing mucous is then swallowed and passes into the stomach via the oesophagus. Cancers of both the stomach and the oesophagus and the large bowel have higher incidences in smokers. Of course the gut and lungs will absorb some of the toxins in cigarettes and these will pass to the liver and kidneys, and from the kidneys to the bladder. All these organs have higher incidences of cancers in smokers.

It is not for this book to tell people to stop any habit, but if they do not wish to increase their illness, or wish to accelerate the recovery, one way is to remove factors that may be making it worse!

Physical agents – radiation, magnets and cycles

Much has been made of the effects of ionizing radiation from nuclear tests and power-station leaks, but there are other possible sources of physical loads such as magnetic fields. Research continues to see whether 'clusters' of cancer outbreaks can truly be associated with living close to power cables. It may be a much more complicated story – perhaps people who have been born near the power lines are better suited to living in that environment than in a different electric field? Are electric blankets creating dangerous fields, for example, since body defences are low at night? Much work could yet be done.

Magnetic bracelets have been pushed hard as a therapeutic tool but it is open to question whether it is appropriate to impose a strong magnetic field on the body twenty-four hours a day. I met one patient who complained of persistent abdominal pain near his appendix. The pain had begun about two months after he began to wear a strong magnetic bracelet on his right wrist. At night, he slept with his wrist very close to the source of pain. A month after removing the bracelet his pain had gone.

Our bodies work in cycles (diurnal, lunar) and maybe the forcing of strong magnetic or electric fields is not a good idea. If someone is already ill it may be best to avoid strong fields. When I first tried to buy a meter to measure electromagnetic fields fifteen years ago, the price in the UK was very high (around £1,500 then!). At that time I could buy the same meter in the US for $200. The market there was larger and the growing user group was that of the 'realtors': estate agents. They had come under increasing pressure to check that houses were elecromagnetically 'safe'.

Sunlight is a powerful source of physical radiation. The combination of increased holidaying in hot climates, together with stronger sunlight, is not good for immunity. Strong sunlight alone has been shown to decrease immunity. Someone recuperating after a serious illness ought *not* to head straight for the fleshpots to cook themselves in the sun! Computers and mobile phones may yet be found to be hazardous. Measures can be adopted to reduce the risk.

Mental stress and the immune system

The events that we experience as 'stress' are very numerous and varied. They include both physical and psychological experiences. Under stress, the performance of our systems alters markedly, usually for the worse. If you can remove or reduce the factors that cause stress, the body can often tackle illness unaided in other ways.

During the vast majority of human history – that is in prehistory – our ancestors hunted or fought in brief spells of high activity, alternating with longer periods of rest. Even activities like grinding corn, although physically hard work, involved little cerebral stress. In contrast, our present lives involve an almost constant need for 'survival' levels of stress. There is almost no balance between high stress and relaxation. There is huge pressure on children to produce good school and university results. There is great emphasis on the rapid acquisition of money and material goods.

Even relaxation has become a highly 'stressful' activity and 'leisure' has become almost as stressful as work. Very few sports remain that do not have a professional component and those who take part commonly aspire to the standards and style set by the leading professional players.

Some time before cancer cells appear in the body, a 'field change' takes place which is a bit like the preparation of a seed-bed before the seeds can grow. This is most easily thought of as an electrical field change. Mental stress, especially prolonged stress, can be one cause of such a field change, allowing other agents to cause damage more easily. Among all the factors that can reduce the effectiveness of the immune system – infectious illness, toxicity, diet, smoking – mental stress can play a major part.

'Depression' – chicken or egg?

Stress can often manifest itself as 'depression'. Depression can be both a result of stress and at the same time a further cause of it. Recent studies have shown that depression can lead to a general increase in many other illnesses. Since depression, along with other manifestations of stress, can seriously damage the immune system, *finding its root cause* is crucial. Searching back from its first onset may yield clues. For example, one of the commonest triggers of depression I have encountered is unresolved bereavement. I will suggest just one example of an exercise to help with bereavement on pages 74–5.

Whether you feel at risk of cancer, or are indeed a cancer patient, the best change you can make to your life is to reduce or avoid stress. People who have settled for a particular style of life tend to accept it, however stressful it may be. They reassess their life choices only if they encounter unexpected change. They may be made redundant or some disaster may crop up in their lives, making it impossible for them to continue their existing plan. I believe that people who use a major crisis to review their life choice and who then select or create a path *which suits them better* will find their health improve.

And if, in addition to this, you can manage to reduce the load of toxicity in your immediate environment, you have already made a significant start in reducing the risks of cancer and improving your chances of recovery from it. Trying to avoid any stresses will help a recovery happen. To try to continue your hard job and lifestyle whilst under-going treatment is like trying to drive with the handbrake on – pointless! Sometimes, the interruptions of routine brought about by necessary hospital visits as part of treat-ment (e.g. outpatients) can be the only 'permissable' way for patients to have a break!

These are just a few of the ways to avoid making things worse. In the next chapter we look at ways of giving the patient more control at the moment of diagnosis and during treatment.

Chapter 2
The Patient's Dilemma

How to handle diagnosis and treatment

The patient's dilemma is this. You have the illness, but the doctor 'officially' has *knowledge*! How do you make these two meet with the best result for yourself?

Part of the purpose of this book is to help you realize how much there is that you can do for yourself outside mainstream medical treatment. You are not, therefore, dependent only on the profession for your recovery. None the less, your doctor will probably play a key role in your treatment and recovery, and in this chapter I hope to make it easier for patients to understand fully what the doctor is saying, and how to respond to it.

The moment of diagnosis

One of the most frightening stages of cancer is the initial diagnosis. A white-coated doctor in formal surroundings often gives the diagnosis and this can, in itself, be intimidating. At such an unsettled time patients, and their families and friends, are often desperate and cling to any life belt. One of the first things that patients seek is firm information. Characteristically they ask:

- What are my chances of recovery?

- If you don't think I will recover, how long will I live?

- How much pain can I anticipate?

These three questions are almost impossible to answer precisely. So the doctor, in order to be as informative and accurate as possible, will normally fall back on statistics.

Understanding the statistics

'Five-year survival' rates

Statistics for cancers are commonly presented in terms of a 'five-year survival rate'. For example, in any particular cancer somebody might be told that there is a '40-per cent five-year survival rate'. This means that if patients are followed up five years from the time of diagnosis, 40 per cent will still be alive. Five years is often considered a

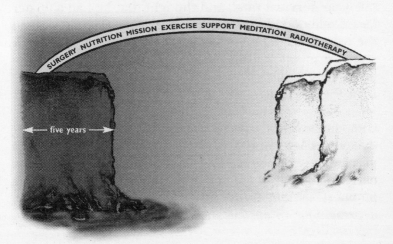

hurdle that, once cleared, leads to an indefinite life span – in other words to 'recovery'.

At the time of diagnosis, the statistics may be explained to the patient or the family. But the circumstances are very stressful and it may be difficult to comprehend fully the implications. People tend to hear only the words 'five years' and assume that their best possible outcome is five more years. Frequently, patients have told me that they expect to drop dead once they've reached five years because they have done their five-year 'best possible outcome'! If they have been given a '40-per cent five-year survival rate' they feel that only 40 per cent of them were 'meant' to survive even that long! The luckless 60 per cent, like lemmings dropping off a cliff, suddenly expect to drop dead at five years and a day in order to fulfil the statistics!

Some time ago I saw a patient shortly after he had been diagnosed with one of the less serious cancers and was surprised that he seemed completely shattered. Then I discovered that he had misunderstood the '95-per cent five-year survival rate', and thought that he had a 95-per cent likelihood of *dying* within five years. Bearing in mind the role of the immune system, and the effects of shock and stress on it, this was an extremely unfortunate misunderstanding.

At the first diagnosis, many patients or their families leave the doctor's surgery in a state of shock. Their shock is compounded by a vague understanding that they have only five years left, and a low chance even of that if the percentage rate sounds low. That is the feeling that many carry home with them. It is a very tough moment – and a *moment which itself can worsen their decline by depressing their system still further.*

'Outcomes' or 'response rates'?

Most doctors are uncomfortable having to impart bad news and the pressure is on them to say what they can do to improve the situation. Enter a second batch of statistics, based on the likely 'outcomes' of surgery, radiotherapy and chemotherapy!

Especially at a time of shock, these statistics too can be confusing. In chemotherapy and radiotherapy, for example, the statistics may state that there is a 'successful response rate' in 70 per cent of tumours. This sounds encouraging. Patients may be persuaded immediately to sign on the dotted line and agree to treatment in the hope that this decision might restore them to the rails they left half an hour ago when they first received the unwelcome news. However, a 'response rate' can mean merely a 'reduction in tumour size' and the reduction in size is often temporary. Of course, when the 'response rate' is first quoted, it is easy to suppose that *responding* means *recovery*. This may be misleading.

At this stage another batch of statistics turns up on the comparative response rates for chemotherapy, radiotherapy and surgery. Then, to confuse the issue still further, response rates are given for *combinations* of these treatments or, even more confusing, for different combinations used at different times in different orders! In a disease category as varied as the cancers, an 'evidence-based' approach to treatment becomes extremely difficult.

Are the statistics applicable to you?

But do all these response rates and outcomes have direct relevance to you? Let's complicate the position still further.

Let's introduce the 'normal distribution curve'. This is the famous bell-shaped curve on a graph that more or less summarizes the fact that common things are commonest. The curve shows that most people bunch around the average and that the rarer an event is the fewer people experience it. But the curve *is* a curve, not a straight line, and everybody occupies a slightly different place on it. In effect, *everybody is unique*. Each individual will occupy a specific place on the curve of whatever is being measured; just because someone has average weight does not mean they are an average height!

This means that you are unique; your response will be unique and your five-year survival will be unique. Don't let the statistics tell you otherwise. If the curve is for treatment responses, remember that it is likely to be for only one form of treatment. There is much else you can do, especially if you accept that you are not 'typical'!

Statistics are a tool for the profession. They are not a prediction of what will happen to you.

So if you are diagnosed with a cancer, or if this happens to a friend or relative, don't be daunted either by the diagnosis or the statistics. First, get the doctor to repeat the essence of what he has said and, if any of the terminology is obscure, ask what they mean. Once you are sure you understand exactly what your doctor has said, maybe you can ask questions – but ask useful ones:

- Your doctor is not necessarily the last medical port of call. There may be other specialists in your illness, or special units or clinics. Ask your doctor who else can help advise you on your illness.

- It greatly helps to talk to others who have had – and

survived – your illness. You can ask your doctor to put you in touch with someone of this kind.

- There are many support organizations for specific types of cancers. Ask your doctor about getting in touch with one.

- You may be able to search the Internet for information or contacts to help you.

- You can also ask your doctor to put you in touch with someone who has had the treatment he is prescribing.

- He should also be able to provide 'five-year outcome improvement' results for that treatment.

- Ask him what side effects you can anticipate, and how to avoid or ameliorate them.

- Lastly, you can ask your doctor if he would take the treatment himself or give it to his family!

You can resolve the patient's dilemma in the same way that you will resolve the other problems associated with your illness – by taking control. Do not be crushed by the moment of diagnosis. Insist on understanding what your doctor is saying, especially the implications of the statistics. Your illness is *your* illness – not any other of the thousands that make up the figures. Once the initial shock of the diagnosis has worn off, you may find an appointment more useful.

And, as subsequent chapters will show you, you can affect your outcome by your own efforts.

Chapter 3
Planning Success

Mental approaches to help recovery

1. The background

Dennis Burkett, famous for Burkett's lymphoma and the high-fibre diet, gave a lecture when I was in medical school on the value of high-fibre diets. Cartoons drawn by his young daughter illustrated the lecture. One of the most memorable was of a wash-basin overflowing, the taps turned full on, and a number of doctors in white coats mopping up the water on the floor. As he said during the lecture, the focus of modern medicine has been to mop up the water rather than turn off the taps – what I call 'salvage medicine'.

But if we look at the 'taps' for cancer, we may well find ways of reducing the flow, or even cutting it off entirely. Professor Burkett ably demonstrated, with the help of those cartoons, that high-fibre diets could dramatically reduce the risk of colon cancers. First-generation Africans in the US, for example, had an incidence of colon cancer 100 times greater than their parents because their parents were eating high-fibre 'natural' foods. A simple enough finding to grasp, perhaps, but one which was not only resisted but disbelieved at first – an astonishing response to such a straightforward statement from a fine and learned man!

So let's start with what might have turned on the taps.

'Triggers' for illness

It is common when taking a full medical history to ask what particular complaint brings the patient to the doctor, and to ask when it began – the 'history of the presenting complaint'. That allows the patient to recall when he first became *aware* of a problem. In the last fifteen years I have increasingly chosen to look back beyond the time when a patient first 'became aware', to uncover any emotional or other stresses that may have led to illness, or to a predisposition to illness.

There is great value in *identifying triggers* that may have weakened the immune system, thereby contributing to a cancer or other serious illness. The most common triggers come under the various headings of 'stress', discussed in the previous chapter.

Healing old wounds

Mental strain, in particular, can trigger serious illness. Up to a point, *physical* strains seem to be self-limiting. In our hunter-gatherer days we knew that after a hard day's exertion we would have to lie down and sleep. The problem with *mental* strain is that it continues to be churned over during sleep, sometimes preventing sleep or leading to early waking. Because these triggers arise from unresolved problems, they can keep nagging the system like a constant strain, indefinitely, until something is done to help resolve them or until the worrier becomes ill.

At this stage some attempt must be made to 'turn off the taps' of the stress. Common causes of stress are bereavement, anger, sadness, fear and abuse. Counselling may provide some alleviation of stress but, in my experience, 'counselling' in serious illnesses, especially in cancers, is a special skill. It not only needs to help people *understand* the causes of unresolved stress. It also needs to *equip them with a number of tools to help resolve, and therefore reduce, the strain of unresolved problems in the past and present*. For example, there are some wonderful tools to deal with sadness and there are some useful tools to deal with bereavement (a common possible cause of sufficient strain to allow a cancer to form). Unsettled or ungrieved bereavement can be one of those loads which nags for years. There are exercises that can greatly help relieve the strain of this. If the loads are left untackled, I believe that all other treatments have much less chance of success. The converse is that, if these problems are sorted, chances of success are far better.

To offer only a tangible, 'body' treatment for a serious illness – without some attempt to address the underlying causes – not only reduces the chances of success, but also wastes an invaluable opportunity for the patient actually to benefit from an unpleasant serious illness. Patients must recognize that stress is the result of their own experience of events rather than a generality that 'just happens' to everybody. We are all exposed to a large number of different strains and stresses. How these affect us depends on the convergence of our genetic code, our upbringing and other factors.

Denial intensifies stress

If you deny your feelings, or try to avoid them by ignoring them or thrusting them to a distance, the causes of stress will never be tackled or resolved. There is little point in driving a car while choosing to ignore a flat tyre or loud noise in the engine.

Disowning the feelings blocks a solution – the 'politician's way'!

A curious English technique in evading difficulties is to 'third party' them. This is a form of denial. People describe how 'one' feels about something – instead of owning it as their *own* feeling. It sounds so peculiar to hear someone say, 'When one moves one's neck one feels sore.' So much easier to say 'When I move my neck, it hurts'! 'I', rather than 'one', can be helped! It would sound pretty odd to hear a doctor say: 'How is one today?' although I have done that to a patient to illustrate the point! If people accept the impact of something on them and their own feelings then solutions can be found.

Another way of 'disowning' feelings is to say that 'when *you* do . . . *you* find . . .' If the patient adopts this manner he is not facing up to his feelings, or to the impact that some event has had on them. Unless they accept the problem as their own, not 'yours', they cannot solve it. Much better for them to say 'when I find . . . I feel . . .' than to say 'when 'one', or 'you' finds . . . and feels . . .'

Once people admit their feelings, something can be done about them.

Distant triggers – reactivating old sores

A relatively small, recent event can open a can of worms from a much more painful moment in the past. For example, going to the funeral of someone who you hardly know can touch on a bereavement which was painful to you – *but not 'dealt with' at the time* – perhaps many years earlier. Films, books and plays can open previous emotional memories. Memory files can be opened very unexpectedly – but not all memories are painful!

I remember going to revise for my surgical exams on a beautiful day in St James's Park in London. After some hard revision, I fell asleep under a tree. When I woke up, I was looking up through the leaves of the tree as they moved gently in the breeze against the blue sky. Suddenly, I had an almost electrical experience as whole chunks of childhood memory were reopened to me. I did not realize what had triggered this until I looked at the label on the tree trunk. I saw that it was a tulip tree – exactly the type of tree (and leaf movement) which I had been parked under in my pram as an infant! The actions of the leaves must have been stored in my brain and, in a way similar to hypnosis, had stimulated access to past memories. This small moment had opened much childhood memory for me. Such moments, places, people and smells could do the same for others. If the memories stirred are happy ones, fine. If they are painful and make a heavy impact then they need to be dealt with or else their impact over time could generate illness.

Serious emotional disturbance and stress, both present and from the past, can affect the onset and development of illness. If you are honest with yourself about your feelings, and take steps to resolve the problems that cause stress or emotional upset, you can reduce the likelihood of illness, and improve your chances of a good outcome if an illness has already happened.

Mental approaches to illness

2. Changes and choices

At the moment of receiving the diagnosis in the doctor's surgery, people feel very vulnerable. They may be confused by the prognosis and many people remain in a shocked and frightened state for some time. I remember one patient who had been told his diagnosis a week before I saw him. He was shaking and unable to speak until I pointed out that many things could be done to help him. I hope that those of you who read on will realize that there is much you can do to improve your own outcome. Once you accept that almost everybody, including yourself, is available as a 'resource', and that it is not only doctors who have the power to grant you a survival ticket, it becomes a question of where to start to plan your future.

You are your own best therapy

One of the most difficult problems for people who live ordered lives is to be thrust into circumstances over which they feel they have no control. It is as if they are in an airliner and suddenly find that the crew has jumped off. In contrast, there is an enormous amount patients can do for themselves over their own bodies – they may even learn to control aspects of their bodies for the first time in their lives if they choose to take an active part in their own recovery.

I have seen many patients who are powerful 'boardroom' corporate individuals. Frequently they try to apply their business methods to sort out their illness, perhaps 'delegating' the problem by paying large sums for 'the best specialist'. They are shocked when that is not enough. One patient said he had been to 'the best surgeons' and had the 'most expensive chemotherapy' and was surprised that this did not appear to be working. When I suggested that the most powerful tool at his disposal lay in the man he saw in the mirror each day, he was surprised. But he did what he needed to and overcame this hurdle. He learned to use the man he saw in the mirror!

A battle or a game of chess?

Corporate minds like the 'hard game', too! Obituaries frequently mention that somebody *fought* cancer, or bravely fought *against* cancer or died after a long *battle* with cancer. I hope that during the course of this book you will learn to see the engagement with illness more as a game of chess than a combat situation. You make one move and your body and mind make another. Your reaction in this case is more dynamic and active than putting up a wall of aggressive obstinacy simply because you think you should *fight* the cancer. In my experience, many of those who take an aggressive, fighting attitude towards their cancers rely on formidable energy and impressive stamina. But they become like a missile without direction and discover that 'missile behaviour' is not enough – they need more elegant tools. If they take an aggressive stance against their cancer then they are, in effect, *attacking themselves*.

I saw one patient who, for several reasons, was destroying himself with anger. He had been made redundant – he thought, unfairly. Not only was he angry about that, but he rapidly became angry about the cancer which had also 'attacked' him. Once he was able to recognize that his anger was destructive he was able to focus on what he *did* want rather than what he did *not* want. For him I recommended the quick anger exercise on pages 72–4. Not only did he have an excellent response but the exercise so amused him that he was moved to teach it to others!

A chance to change

I remember facing a depressed group of cancer patients at the cancer help centre one day and I wanted to inject a little energy into the group (a car that is stationary cannot be steered!). I thought I would throw a verbal 'hand grenade' among them, so I told them that they were lucky! Disbelief showed on almost every face. I told them that they could be regarded as lucky because they had not been hit by a bus that morning and still had some choice over their outcome! A lively discussion followed. But they were not dead, and they still had a choice.

In the past it was held that illness was not so much an abnormality but a much more 'normal' feature of the cycles of life. But drugs and medical techniques have become so powerful, and lives so demanding, that we expect few people to suffer illness for long. Illness is often regarded now as merely an inconvenience in our lives quickly to be overcome by the available technological weaponry. We can then revert to 'normal life' again.

It helps patients to put aside this expectation and to regard illness as a 'wake-up call'. When illness strikes, they can take stock of their situation and see if there is any

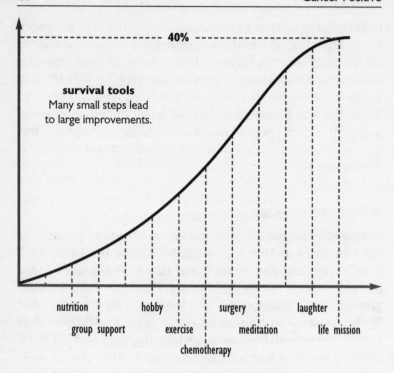

survival tools
Many small steps lead
to large improvements.

40%

nutrition · group · support · hobby · exercise · chemotherapy · surgery · meditation · laughter · life · mission

change that might make their lives healthier and more enjoyable – even if the illness dramatically disappears. In other words it is an opportunity to look for a *change in life direction*, or a *different perspective*.

Choosing a healthier life

Like unemployment, illness can be an opportunity to make new and useful choices. We'll look at some ways of doing this later in the book. But to make the best of change, people need to have a clear idea of what they would really like to do with their lives, and how to make productive choices at each step along the way. Certainly, to treat the physical symptoms only to return to the stressful life that led up to the illness is pointless.

'Life choice' time?

Illness can raise the fundamental question – what is your 'life mission'. To make the choice of an exciting and stimulating future could be at least enjoyable and might even save your life- in many different ways. This is infinitely healthier than merely continuing a career of only mild interest, clinging to it because you have always done it or because there is a secure income (what good is that if you do not live to spend it?) or because others might be affected if it was given up. With an appropriate use of the tools that I'll introduce later, a number of people have stated that their illness turned out to have been one of the most 'enriching' experiences that they'd had. In some cases they said that they were grateful because they had the opportunity to take stock and make changes, finally 'living' rather than 'enduring' life.

Avoiding the 'sympathy trap'

The 'sympathy trap' occurs when people with a serious illness find that others flock around to *sympathize* with them. Sympathy may seem attractive and welcome, but it doesn't do much to encourage you to move on from your illness. Sympathy leaves you where you are – it is a poor 'strategy'. Assistance, support and guidance are far better gifts than sympathy.

I recall one patient who became sick with rheumatoid arthritis and the whole family tree, and others, arrived to pay homage. When she retired to her bed; many 'long-lost' relatives emerged and flowers arrived by the lorryload. She was the centre of attention and it was the best time she had ever had. But there was no advantage that she could see in getting better! I pointed out to her that the 'attention' path might kill her but she 'milked it' for a couple more weeks. Soon she became bored with sympathy and flowers and began to worry that she might die without leaving her bed. I pointed out that she could get attention and gifts in many other ways that were less dangerous!

She shed the bitterness of her past, chose a new path for her future and left her bed. She began to improve, became mobile again and lived several years more, happier than she had ever been when dependent on others.

The pitfall of the 'search-for-sympathy' strategy is that your short-term needs are better served by the illness than by being well again. Clearly, if you have begun to enjoy sympathy (as opposed to supportive attention and energy) it can have a detrimental effect on your outcome.

The daily cycle of stress – give maintenance a chance

In the daily hormonal 'dip' following a midday meal, it is not at all uncommon to become sleepy. In hunter-gatherer days, that is probably exactly what we did. However, anybody caught having an afternoon nap in today's high striving culture might be looked down on. We no longer pursue a wide range of daily activities, but tend instead to specialize in a few, with a consequent increase in stress. If the demands of the daily schedule are too persistent then the body's engine is simply racing all the time, with no opportunity for maintenance and repair. I believe there is value in re-instituting a *range* of daily activities so that there is at least a balance. It is essential to allow some quiet time for the repair and maintenance processes to function.

For some people, the only solitude they can find happens in the daily commute in their car. Now the mobile phone may have invaded even that!

In my younger days I was an international oarsman. We trained enormously hard but we also ate and slept. I do not believe we would have achieved as much had we trained more and rested less. Just as you must train to be fit, so you must also balance that with time to relax and recuperate.

How to relax

Relaxation can be passive or active. You can sit, lie, sunbathe or snooze, or you can take exercise, pursue a hobby or generally enjoy yourself. Relaxation can take many forms. For some, hobbies produce a relaxed state. I used to enjoy woodcarving, whilst listening to the radio. Some people enjoy listening to music and some enjoy sailing boats. Each will know what relaxes them.

Relaxation or meditation?

Unfortunately the word 'meditation' can conjure up a 'knit-your-own-yoghurt' society for some people, complete with beads, headbands and dope! Moreover, the bookshelves are full of books on how to meditate 'in the right way'. As with medical treatment, I think the 'right way' is the one that works for you. Most people will find through experiment a way that works for them.

During meditation, the body's repair processes can take place, and the *range* of the body's physiological ability can be relearned. The immune system has an opportunity to regenerate and to consider the challenges that have been sent to it that day or over previous weeks or months. Food can be digested, and more value can be squeezed out of the opportunity simply to stop. The body and mind can then be prepared for the next challenge.

A hobby may be an admirable form of relaxation, but it is not the same as meditation. In *relaxing*, the body aims at a reduced level of constant mental drive. In *meditation* the aim is to create a mental 'vacuum' in which there is no active, conscious thought – the Buddhist 'void'. This is not easy. As with a sport, you cannot expect to be an expert at the end of the first day. Even a fortnight's holiday is sometimes not enough for ordinary relaxation to take place, let alone meditation.

An almost 'monastic' peace is a good ambience for meditation and it is well worth creating a quiet place and time at home. That normally means early or late hours. The early hours of the morning are often particularly valuable because the process can then set up the body (and mind) for the rest of the day.

New challenges

Exciting things can happen when you learn new techniques. To take up meditation can entirely change your view of life. It can make you aware of your ability to make choices about your bodily and mental processes, and the results are long-lasting. It is not possible to become 'unaware' again. People taking part in this 'awareness' tend to collect around them other people who are 'waking up' at the same time. New directions and interests can be challenging to relations or friends. Some of your friends and relations will support you, but others may find it difficult.

Meditation could even help you replace your old, inflexible mental approach to your body with new, more flexible ideas and attitudes. As I said at the beginning of this section, you are your own best therapy. It is in your power to make changes and choices that can improve your health. These can be straightforward physical options – like exercise and diet – or fundamental changes to your mental state – like eliminating stress, spotting and avoiding the sources of stress, and adopting a therapy, like meditation, that can transform your mental approach to your whole mind and body.

In short, a serious illness can often be an opportunity that jolts you out of your rut and presents you with new opportunities.

Mental approaches to 'wellness'

3. Looking ahead – how to begin

There is not much point stepping into a car without a destination in mind – unless your aim is just to enjoy driving. If you do know where you want to go then the first step is to plan how to get there. If you haven't been there before you might use a map or ask someone who knows the way.

In the same way, recovery from illness is improved if there is a worthwhile and well-defined aim to be achieved by recovering. Recovery is greatly assisted if it is not an end in itself but merely a stage to some greater end. If you have

a clear objective then you have a much better chance of
attaining it. Also, a clear forward focus will distract you
from looking all the time at what you are *trying to avoid*
(remember the illness?). If you are driving at night it is
important not to look at the lights of the car coming towards
you! It's equally unhelpful to try to drive forwards by looking
only in the rear view mirror, looking at where you have been
in the hope that this will guide you to the road ahead!

'Knowing' where to go

Racing drivers tend to look not at the *next* corner or
obstacle but *beyond* it. The metaphor is valuable for health.
I like to find out what my patients want to do with their
lives. When I ask whether they want to recover or whether
they wish to live the response is usually: 'Well, *of course* I
would like to recover'. If this question is followed up with
'Why?' or 'What for?' it is frequently followed by silence or
confusion. Some muted responses include statements like:
'Well I want to get back to . . .'

Of course the significance of '*back* to' is this; their life
before they became ill *was contributing to the illness in
the first place*. So to aim to return to that state *without any
alteration* is unlikely to be helpful. In fact it is like
returning to a dangerous addiction. Rewinding the tape to
where it was does not change the film's outcome.

Even the worst situation can be improved

I can remember starting a new surgical job and inheriting a
number of patients who had feet in an advanced state of
gangrene. I couldn't see that these 'long-dead' feet could
possibly be rescued. One of the patients had even been in

hospital for fourteen months watching one toe after another disappear, and watching the gangrene slowly but surely creep up his leg. My feeling was that these feet would have to be removed in order to restore the health of the patient and to give them the opportunity to restart a lifestyle.

It would have been classic old-fashioned dictatorial surgery to say: 'What you need is an amputation'. But I was in my first week in the job, and I thought a number of immediate amputations might threaten future patient intakes!

I approached each of the patients in turn and asked them what they wanted from their lives, offering them a number of different options. Maybe some of them wanted to stay in hospital whilst others wanted to go home. Maybe some were happy to be in a wheelchair whilst others wanted to walk again. Maybe some wanted to be able to walk on crutches whilst others wanted to be equipped with an artificial leg. I merely put it to them that it would be helpful to me if they made a decision about what they *wanted from their lives*. Then I would do my best to pull in the resources available to them. I explained that, although an amputation led to a 'loss' of part of them, the amputation would remove a foot that was *not* working and replace it with one that *did* work. Thus an apparent backward step could turn out to be a major move forward, with all the new possibilities which could unfold for them. A *loss* of a limb became a *gain* of mobility.

I did not look for immediate responses from the patients. I arranged in some cases for previous amputees to visit them. Within a few days two patients had decided to have amputations. One of them was happy to be able to live in a wheelchair at home. The other one wanted an artificial leg after he had spoken with another patient who had had a below-knee amputation and was still playing squash successfully! After those two patients had had the amputation the others saw the improvement in their morale and physical health and opted for the operation themselves.

The result was that a focused group of patients used their illness as an opportunity to consider what they *really* wanted out of their lives. This must be one of the greatest gifts that an illness can make to an individual. If illness gives you the chance to make choices that you might have made years earlier, but didn't, then the illness has served an important purpose for you, and almost certainly for those around you. Often a patient, suitably awoken and suitably enthusiastic, can become a teacher among his own community. I have had several patients who have said that illness gave them their real purpose in life, as well as a wish to help others.

The absence of a forward plan or target makes it tricky for the body to know what is expected of it. To return to a car analogy – *not* to have a focus is like asking a mechanic to prepare a car for a major journey without telling him what the journey will entail. If you tell him what you need the car for – a desert or an arctic journey – then he can equip it for the task which you have chosen.

What next?

Let us assume that you know you have a serious illness. You have taken the opportunity to review your way of life. You have rearranged your affairs to reduce stress and to avoid the psychological pitfalls that might undermine your positive mental approach to your situation. You have chosen your objective and have planned a route to it, even if your objective is to die peacefully: a clear target in itself for which your strategy can be adjusted accordingly.

These are all 'strategic' considerations. What about 'tactics'? How do you now, in your day to day life, maintain this course?

Your next step must be to plan the day-to-day tactics that will help you pursue a forward path. Of course you can always change the forward path – it doesn't have to be fixed – but the essential feature must be to encourage you to 'aim over the horizon' and not just at the next problem.

There are a number of useful tactics or game plans that can be used to make 'aiming over the horizon' a great deal easier, and in the next chapter I shall look at them in some detail.

Chapter 4
Approaches for Success

1. Helping the doctor help you

As we have seen in a previous chapter, 'going to the doctor' is not a straightforward business of presenting your symptoms and receiving a diagnosis and treatment. If you have a serious illness then your doctor could be one of the most important people around you. At the very least your doctor has access to a system which uses some of the most expensive tools! In this section we look at ways in which you and you doctor can interact to make the best of what that profession has to offer.

It's your future, not the doctor's

Patients tend to look at doctors as the sole arbiters of their fate. Of course, one of the choices available to you *is* to say to the medical profession 'make me better' but this ignores the enormous contribution you can make to your own outcome. You will gain better results if you approach doctors with this mental attitude: 'this is what I believe would help. Please do what you can to help.' You can become a victim of your illness, or you can use it as a signal to make a change for the better. Think of recovery not as going *back* to a previous life, but as going *forward* to a better one.

When I point out to patients that their life before illness, or some part of it, may have contributed to their illness, their reactions vary from disbelief to anger. But once you have realized that your way of life *could be* a factor, it becomes clear that only *you* can plan your future lifestyle. You can draw on support from many quarters, of course, but only *you* will ultimately make the choice of what *you* do.

You are unique – not just a statistic

There's a tendency – especially in Britain – for patients to be 'obedient' and 'reasonable'. They tend to do what they are told and to accept the statistics and to assume that they will fall somewhere along the middle line of the recovery curve.

But will you? You may well be able to use your unique characteristics to buck the statistical trend, and you must not allow statistics to cow you. Time and again people need to be reminded that they are unique. Statistics are a tool for the profession. They should not influence your mental approach to your illness. Remember that blade of grass!

Is there any point asking 'How long, doctor'?

Not much. Everybody is different. Survival rates and outcome rates, even for the same cancer 'labels', vary a lot. The doctor is under great pressure to come up with a definite prognosis, and the patient and family feel desperate to know for 'certain'. In fact there is little certainty, and it is doubtful if a 'minimum and maximum' figure is of much practical or psychological help.

Buck the downward trend!

More important still, asking for a prognosis can become a self-fulfilling prophecy. If you want to believe bad news it is out there. If you want to believe good news it's out there too. At first, everybody died of Aids within a year. As soon as some people started to defy that by being *unreasonable*, more and more people started to survive for longer. There may be the same opportunity for moving the statistics in cancers. As soon as people begin to realize that there is something they can do about it, over and above the routine medical approaches, then the statistics may alter. Otherwise, every time people are told what the statistics are for the normal distribution of the population, they tend obey them and the statistics stay the same!

Breaking the (bad?) news

There is remarkably little training for doctors, even nowadays, in how to present news of illness to patients, how to empathize with their situation or how to deal with the patient's family.

It is at this crucial moment of giving a diagnosis that an enormous amount of damage (or good) can be done. It is one thing to state to a patient: 'Ah yes, you're here to hear the results of the test done last week. I am so sorry – it's bad news.' This blunt approach closes a door on the rest of the conversation unless the patient has the determination to persist in asking questions. A more productive approach may be to say 'There is a challenge ahead and we need to find the best way around it'. Immediately there is a sense that the door is still open.

How not to break news

When I was in Borneo, studying tropical diseases, I remember a cancer diagnosis being given to a patient who had had an excision biopsy of a lump on his tongue. The lump was sent to the laboratory in Singapore for analysis. Having sweated with worry through the week as he waited for the report the patient was summoned to hear the biopsy result and the doctor said: 'Well, it's very simple – you've got cancer.' The doctor might as well have pulled a gun and shot him. An hour later, after we had discussed the information more carefully with him, it began to dawn on him that an excision with 'good margins' didn't necessarily constitute a death penalty! Twenty years later he is still alive. He became highly motivated in helping others.

The Internet

The Internet enables patients to obtain almost limitless 'information' on different tumours and illnesses. However, it is not always easy to make sense of the information on the Internet. Patients occasionally turn up with box files full of information on what they regard as their 'condition'. One of the difficulties is the 'label' of their diagnosis. Has the 'label' been correct, and have they looked up the right words on the search engine? They might have a leiomyoma in their gut and have looked it up under a leiomyosarcoma. In that situation the box file would be useless – and unnecessarily alarming.

There are masses of medical sites on the Internet and they vary enormously. Two of the most informative sites I have seen are those set up by Ralph Moss:

www.ralphmoss.com; www.cancerdecisions.com.

The issue of so-called 'false hope'

To raise 'false hopes' has often been presented as a 'bad thing'. If a patient has been told that he has a serious illness then it is thought irresponsible to encourage unrealistic optimism. Hope can, however, help people recover. In a similar way, dashing a patient's hopes can assist decline. I think that is possibly a worse thing to do – the impact of some people's comments can be like the aboriginal 'pointing of the bone'. In this ritual the witch doctor points a bone at someone who has been sentenced to death. The person it is pointed towards knows what the pointing means and accepts that they will die. Telling someone in a very downbeat way that 'Unfortunately you have cancer' may have a similar effect. Offering some hope can have direct impact on their 'state' and immune system.

If the medical profession could always explain how illness arose in the first place then it would be more convincing when they are so 'certain' about the bad news they pass on. But, nobody, including doctors, can fully explain the mechanism by which cancers arise. That is why they should not dismiss out of hand other chances of recovery, however inexplicable they may seem. The fact is that there are many factors in recovery of which direct physical intervention is but one.

Is there a common factor in people who recover?

When Carol Hirschberg studied her book on 'spontaneous remissions' from cancers and looked at a large number of patients who had recovered from malignancy without any medicines, surgery or chemotherapy, she found some unexpected results. I asked her during dinner at a cancer conference in Holland if she had sensed a common link in those who recovered unexpectedly, without treatment. She told me that those who recovered spontaneously had encountered a 'sense of love'. You can't put that into a bottle and drink it! I feel that the sense of love may have been from, and for others – but also *for the patient themselves*.

Official statistics may give a clue

A Royal Marsden study published in the *Lancet* in October 1987, looking at the value of 'group support' in breast cancer patients, demonstrated powerfully that 'group support' during the year after diagnosis practically doubled the five-year survival rate. If that had been a pharmaceutical drug, imagine the stock market climb for the company making it!

The 'outpatient' problem

Outpatient visits are geared to your prognosis. If you have a slow pattern of cancer, you will be given appointments that are a long way apart – say six months. If it is regarded as a fast-growing cancer then your appointments may be at monthly intervals. This appointment system may contribute to the disease by making you too dependent on your visits (if you hope for permission to live) and deterring you from taking other action. You have the chance to look after yourself and to receive support twenty-four hours a day! Use it!

How to be in your own constant care

When I was a surgeon in a district hospital I inherited an outpatient system based purely on 'time' intervals for follow-up – three months, six months, nine months, or twelve months. If a patient had an outpatient appointment in three months and became ill the day after their appointment, they often did not act because they *already had their next appointment booked*. That left them unsupported until that appointment, when they could have been receiving care immediately.

This system of 'holding on' to patients also jammed the outpatients department – I used to see eighty-five patients in four hours, which did not give them very long! I decided to change the booking procedure for outpatients and stopped 'repeat' visits based purely on time intervals. Instead, I told patients what I would be looking for during their visits and encouraged them to take part in their own care. By examining themselves they could check themselves every day. I wrote to their GPs to suggest what they might also be looking for in case the patients went to see them.

In order to maintain active support for the patients I agreed to see any patient *within a working day* if they were troubled by anything at all and couldn't see their GP. Patients were then supported all the time, empowered to manage their own lives and no longer floating between appointments. In this way, too, the number of patients in the clinics declined dramatically, which meant that when people did turn up for an outpatient appointment there was more time to talk to them.

Don't depend solely on outpatient visits

In a 'timed interval' system patients remain in a state of worry up to their next appointment, leaning too much on the expectation of seeing the doctor – maybe hoping to be 'given permission' to feel well. If patients are given constant follow-up appointments then their focus never comes off their *illness*, because they are constantly being reminded that they *have* an illness. A more interesting and useful form of follow-up is to check on how well each patient is *meeting the objectives for their new life*. In that way their focus would always be *forwards*.

So much for how you can interact with your doctor to achieve the best outcome for yourself. But the help of your doctor, and the facilities he can draw on for you, is just *one* of the day-to-day stratagems you can use to speed your recovery. Other people also play an important role, as we shall see in the next section.

2. Creating a mission

Give yourself a kick start

If you are suffering the shock of an adverse diagnosis or if you are undergoing debilitating treatment then you may have neither the confidence nor the physical inclination to take on a 'mission'. You may feel that any sort of life style 'mission' can wait until your illness is cured.

But the mission is part of the cure, and should not be postponed. A great time to begin enjoying life's good side, joys, friends or hobbies is NOW!

To get yourself going, even when you don't feel like it, decide on your objectives. Then tell that circle of friends

who will make sure, through encouragement, that you stick
to the path you have chosen.

The mission

Have a target! If you have no dream then you cannot make
it happen. At the very least, go through the process of
imagining and exploring what sort of life you would really
like and what helps to concentrate your mind. Frequently,
people have a sense of what they *think* they would like to
do or be, but on closer examination they discover quite
another vocation! But whatever it is, you must have an
objective. Until you have a plan or target, you are not free
because you are waiting for 'life' to deal the next card. If
you have a group of good friends then it is worth asking for
their help by telling them what you would like to achieve.
Such meetings can be enjoyable and can generate all sorts
of solutions. One technique used in ancient Persia was to
have two sets of meetings to solve a problem: one teetotal
and one fortified by wine. The scribes would take notes for
both meetings. More often than not, the solutions provided
at the more 'relaxed' meeting were the ones subsequently
adopted! While I am not advocating alcohol by itself as the
solution to any problem, a relaxed atmosphere certainly
throws up more ideas – and if nothing else, you will have
had a good time!

Do something new – and exciting

I believe that it is important for people, when they are
creating a strategy for their own future, to test something
that is outside their normal routine. The overwhelming
majority of people have learned to live within certain 'safe'

guidelines. Many people will look at the work they have been doing and assume that any new path they will follow must be similar on the basis that it is 'too late to learn something completely new'. But they had to learn their existing job, so why not learn a new one? A state of learning is very exciting, and being around other people who are learning is an added bonus.

Choose an occupation that suits

We have already discussed that a crucial part of any 'beyond recovery' life is to find stimulating activities and interests. Many patients have no idea what they want to do in their lives and find it difficult to make changes to long-established patterns as they grow older. There are many ways in which you can explore choices for your future – perhaps for the first time in your life – to find what really makes you tick.

Some suggestions:

1. Recall a good experience from the past and see if it gives clues about what might excite you now

2. Exploring various hobbies or re-activating one you previously had insufficient time for may help trigger an idea

3. Sometimes activities that bring you within a circle of stimulating friends may be worth looking into

4. Find a list of adult-education courses (e.g. at a local college) and look through it to see if inspiration comes

5. The 'six-month diary' mentioned later might stimulate a process.

Crucially, these new initiatives include company, pastimes or activities that *lift your spirits and which you look forward to doing*.

I remember one patient who was an excellent hobby artist but whose job was pest control. He enjoyed his work, but there came a time when his mobility was restricted by the growth of a lump in his leg. When the lump (benign as it turned out) was removed he moved to Scotland with his wife and began to paint more. He became known for his paintings and sold them in hotels and country clubs. This not only brought him additional income but also gained him recognition for his real skills. He could do as much or as little of the pest control as he chose from that moment. He had found and created a life that suited him.

Saving 'fun' for retirement is often a false economy. For a number of reasons you may not want – or be able – to do your chosen pastime when you reach retirement. One answer is to *do it now*.

Solitude or sociability?

There are excellent solitary activities, but I recommend at the beginning that your new activities involve other people. If you take up woodworking, for example, you may need to become apprenticed to a good 'master' for a time to help you develop your skills. Whatever path you choose, *encouragement is of enormous value*. You need to draw people around you who can make your choice possible. The last thing you want is people who stand around saying: 'You must be crazy, why on earth do you want to do that?'

Avoid 'downers'

A frequent snag when you are trying to develop a new style of life is an associate – or number of associates – who try to hold you back. They may do so for the best reasons – concern for your safety or health – but they will quickly undermine your resolve.

Be ruthless! Avoid 'suppressive' people. You may already know who they will be. They might be the people who, you notice, 'drain' you on the phone or who 'dump' their woes on you when you meet or talk. It is just not helpful to mix with dull groups of people or individuals who are still doing what they always have in life, even when they are unhappy about it. 'Downers' often speak from fear, because they do not want to confront their own limits of understanding. Again, surround yourself with people who are encouraging and enjoyable to be with and in whose company you feel that the whole is greater than the sum of the parts.

Regular 'review'

If you choose your mission when you are at a physical or emotional low ebb, it may subsequently need revision. Never be shy of doing this. I would suggest a regular review of your mission. The support group can act as useful 'leverage' to check that you are up to the mark. It is worth pointing out that support team members can function well on a 'need-to-know' basis. They do not have to know your whole dream – only those parts that you wish them to support. It may well be that your mission is very private but you need help with certain bits. For example, you may wish to visit an indigenous population in a faraway country and need help with airfares or tickets. You may well have someone who can help with those practicalities. They do not need to know why you are flying there. Too much 'sharing' might weaken a mission.

It is fun to have a support team composed of enthusiasts. At any given time, one of them may be the 'lead' enthusiast, but together they can egg each other on. They can also act as your mirror for the mission. In this way, you are drawing on human resources to help you stick to your chosen path. In so doing, your body will 'recognize' your single-mindedness. Once it does this, your body will activate its own internal pharmacy to ensure that it is in the best shape to help achieve your goal.

In the next chapter we deal with a number of practical 'tools' which can be used to help.

3. Creating a support team

Allow other people to help keep you on your chosen path

Don't face your challenges alone. People perform better together. So look on all your family, friends and acquaintances as potential supporters. One of the most difficult challenges for those who have so often helped others is to *learn to accept help themselves*. I firmly believe that just learning to receive can be a powerful contributor to some people's recovery.

As a hospital surgeon I used to explain to patients that I could devote a certain amount for them in the surgery but that they would need to do certain things for themselves. Occasionally we made this into a 'contract', and I encouraged their fellow ward members to help them to keep their side of the contract. This made them realize that by enlisting the support of their friends they were applying 'leverage' to help them achieve their chosen mission. Such support can help patients through even the toughest patches and in the hospital life was often great fun.

Of course your support team can be recruited from among practically everyone you know and meet, not merely your fellow patients.

What sort of team do I need?

The 'right' team depends, of course, on your chosen mission.

Everybody's chosen support team will differ – just as the objective differs. The people and the resources available close to home will vary enormously. It is crucial to create a team that not only matches your objective but also *feels* supportive.

Broadly, most 'support teams' will include one or more people from the following groups.

Medical support

Frequently, one branch of a support team will be a member of the medical profession. This might be your doctor, radiotherapist, surgeon, oncologist or nurse. Often patients strike up a better rapport with nurses and physiotherapists than with doctors, since they have longer contact with them and more chances to talk. Speaking to patients has been a major part of the training of Macmillan nurses, for example.

The resources of the medical profession are *not* the only resources available to patients but they are, possibly, the most *powerful and useful* resources available! So if you co-opt your doctor as a member of your team, you've got access to some heavy artillery. And it also helps to *manage* this relationship. Attend outpatient sessions with information about your other support activities; it makes the doctor aware that you are actively working for yourself. Take the initiative. It is well worth starting the appointment by stating what would work for you. Point out areas where you feel you need help and say: 'Now, this is where I could do with some support. Can you help me?' This makes clear to the doctor what your objectives are, and leaves *you* in the driving seat.

Physical support

Many people enlist the help of non-medical specialists – nutritionists, reflexologists, aromatherapists and counsellors. Who you choose will depend on your needs and habits, and also who lives nearby or who might have been recommended to you. They do not need to live close by; you can always use telephone, email or help. I have often steered patients to a telephone consultation with Ute Brookman (well known at the Bristol Cancer Help Centre) for advice on nutrition. As well as giving nutritional advice on the phone, she will prepare and post supplements. You may never meet some members of your support 'team', but there's no reason why you shouldn't enlist this sort of expertise.

Morale support

In addition to medical and physical support, you could co-opt friends, relations and companions who help you feel well in mind and spirit. Normally, in a family, one person will tend to be outstandingly helpful. Who that person is may change, as the patient's needs change. Often the most helpful members of a family are those who have been through hardship themselves – illness or otherwise. They tend to have a depth of understanding that is learned only by experience. It is difficult to 'train' such understanding, or to absorb it merely by reading about it.

New directions need new team members

If your objectives involve taking up a new hobby or some other fresh initiative then you will find new team members in that occupation *who may be completely unaware and remain unaware that you have any illness*. I knew one patient who had always wanted to learn free fall parachuting but had been putting it off. When a cancer was diagnosed she decided to 'give it a go' – at fifty-seven – and found wonderful support and enthusiasm among the instructors and other students. She told them nothing of her 'illness', as she had chosen to consider it as being 'over'. One of the things she most enjoyed was being amongst younger, motivated and excited people who had in common with her only that they loved the same hobby! She was still parachuting six years later – her focus had shifted from being ill to being excited.

It is important to feel excitement when meeting members of your team and to look forward to the changes that a good support structure will bring about. Not all the members of a team need to know about each other. They are a group of people that you have chosen to help you move from a difficult time to an exciting time that stimulates your mind and therefore also your body.

A good support team will help you move forward to your post-recovery objectives. The members of a team can be changed at any time. Once you have formed your support structure it is remarkable how quickly the excitement of new challenges pushes the thought of illness into the background. Moreover, you will find that you become an inspiration to others, thus attracting around you other inspired people.

Summary

- Decide what you want to achieve

- Decide what help you need to make it happen best

- Choose a team that would best help – and is fun

- Start moving forwards

- Review the mission

Chapter 5
Some Practical Tools for Success

We've dealt with the strategy and tactics of success – the general plan and the day-to-day management of it. Now I would like to give you some 'tools' for success – all the techniques and devices that will keep your mind dynamic, working to influence your body to get better. Some of them are the slightest of tricks – like trying not to smile – while some are serious disciplines. Some may seem strange coming from an 'orthodox' doctor, but even if only one works this book will have been worth it!

Flying through clouds

In a light aircraft, when the weather worsens, it can look pretty tough below the clouds. Indeed a significant number of accidents happen when pilots allow themselves to be forced lower by cloud, possibly ending up in a mountain-side which they could not see because of bad weather. Choices of what they might do include continuing in bad weather, landing, or flying higher (probably with the help of a radar controller). Flying higher often means flying through cloud until the aircraft emerges into bright sunshine. A whole new perspective arrives with the clear sky – a horizon is visible, the air is still and there is no ice – and the pilot will be able to see any hills or mountains ahead of him.

This could be a metaphor for illness. When difficulties arise, some people just press on without a change of direction. That approach might work but is likely, in a worsening situation, to lead to trouble. To seek help and to climb through cloud is similar to seeking help in an illness – maybe from a doctor or friend – to guide you to a situation where you regain control for yourself. You can then equip yourself to fly to a safer situation and land safely. At the very least, you have created an opportunity for helpful solutions to happen – and have taken charge of the situation yourself.

Posture – even standing up straight might help

Adjusting your posture can be very useful. Your body is always with you, and you can practise helpful posture at any time, wherever you are. At difficult times it is helpful to stand tall, with chest out, head back and feet a shoulder's width apart to provide a stable base. In this position, decisions that you make are more likely to be helpful, it is easier to receive challenging news and it is easier to cope on the telephone. The converse – to stand slumped with head down and shoulders forward – brings people into a low 'state'. Although adjusting posture may seem a bit trite and simple it can be highly effective.

If you feel a spell of low morale or gloom coming on then stand in the 'stable position' (as above) and lift your arms up and outstretched to a position a bit beyond vertical. This can help to ward off a spell of depression. Furthermore, to have good posture helps with most of the other exercises described here.

The lemon-juice visualization test

I have already briefly described 'the lemon-juice visual-ization' test. I'm going to give it now in its entirety to demonstrate just how well it works and to dispel any lingering scepticism among those who don't accept that the mind can significantly affect the body's functions. It is vital to your recovery that you *know* that your state strongly influences the functions of your body.

This test is best done in a quiet room with people sitting in ordinary chairs, feet firmly on the floor and with their eyes closed. Hands and feet should not be crossed. The gathering should be invited to imagine – to visualize – the following story.

Imagine that you're in the desert. Imagine that it's hot. You can feel the heat beating down. You've been walking for several hours. It is around mid-morning. The sun is approaching its height and you can feel the heat beating up off the sand. You can see the heat shimmering. You can feel the dry, dusty sand in your shoes, in your clothes and in your hair. The sand has also mixed with the sweat on your face so you can feel the dryness. Your lips are dry, your mouth is dry and you are just approaching town where you will be spending the rest of the day. You are looking forward to a shower, a cool drink and a chance to shed this overall dusty, dry feeling.

Just before you reach the town with all its possible luxuries, you approach a lemonade stall, rather like the ones they have in the United States, which is being manned by a young boy. It is a shaded stall with an umbrella protecting it from the heat of the sun. Just as you draw level with the stall the young boy gestures for you to stop, opens the lid on the insulated trolley and takes out a metal plate on which there are lemon segments separated by ice cubes. He offers you one of the lemon segments. You take it off the tray and you place it on your tongue. You notice how it feels, how cold it is. You notice the feeling in your mouth. You notice how sharp the lemon is. You enjoy the feeling of having a piece of juicy, cool lemon sitting on your tongue. After a moment of savouring the lemon, courage gets the better of you and you sink your teeth into the lemon segment. Notice how it feels – the sharp taste of the lemon, the coolness of the lemon juice. You savour the taste, enjoying for a moment the refreshing feeling of the lemon segment in your mouth. Having squeezed the last drops from the lemon segment you remove the skin from your mouth and place it in the bin that the boy has been holding for you. You then prepare to cover the last short distance into the town.'

At this stage, the 'sitters' can be encouraged to be aware of the floor under their feet and to 're-enter' the room and open their eyes. Asked if they noticed anything, they will frequently say: 'Yes. Increased salivation in the mouth.' Point out that this is purely the result of a thought based on fiction and past experience. The lemon slice did not exist. The process by which thought causes salivation is a complicated one involving several nerve connections, and the production and release of special liquid from three groups of salivary glands.

It is no very great leap from appreciating this to under-standing how a long term thought or feeling could have long term effects on your body. The lemon-juice exercise is extremely short-lived. Prolonged and stressful thought could have a much greater impact on the body, especially when spread over many years.

There is also an added bonus to this test. If you did have an increase in salivation because of the test, you have shown that you can successfully 'visualize', and visualization is a great help in many other exercises that will speed your recovery.

Shedding the haversack of anger – The CAT'S TEETH!

For anyone with a serious illness anger is an unnecessary burden – like a haversack full of bricks. Amongst many other areas anger adversely affects the immune system, blood pressure and heart beat. It is relatively straight-forward to offload and this exercise ought to be considered before any of the others. Once the anger is out of the way the other exercises will be done much better.

Anger and sadness are often linked and tend to congregate in the upper part of the chest. Sobbing and 'being uptight' both happen at the top of the chest. Laughter happens at the bottom of the chest. Anger is concentrated at what is called, in Hindu medicine, the throat 'chakra', and it is useful to make use of the throat chakra to offload anger.

In Hindu medicine, the body contains different 'chakras' or 'energy centres' of the body. In most common descriptions, seven chakras are described – crown, brow, throat, heart, stomach, spleen and base. Different chakras denote different types of energy and the throat is associated with expression.

When people are angry they sometimes express or 'shed' part of it by shouting at each other. Unfortunately, too often this is superficial shouting without real clarity. Other techniques for shedding anger, such as 'effigy bashing' or beating a mattress with a tennis racket, may be good extra tools but they fail to use that useful route nature has given us – our voices.

By using the throat chakra as an outlet for anger you can help to purge yourself of it. Of course it is not very English to express feelings, let alone make a noise! Now you can do so – with good reason! Imagine how many fights might not happen if people used a 'safe' way of offloading their anger! The benefits of fifteen seconds of anger release far outweigh any disadvantage caused by raising the eyebrows of neighbours or other listeners! The following exercise – using the throat chakra – is the best I have yet encountered for shedding anger.

The Cat's-Teeth exercise

It's up to you where you do this exercise, but out in the open is great. Your own house is fine (someone else's house might be even better!). If you are doing this within possible earshot of neighbours remember to clap loudly when you have finished. This will reassure them that it was a performance!

For this fifteen-second exercise, stand squarely with your feet about a shoulder's width apart. Imagine whoever or whatever most easily resurrects your anger standing about four metres in front of you. Imagine a cat on their right.

Then, using the index finger of your right hand, the 'Mars' finger (if you are left handed, use your left 'Mars' finger, and imagine the cat on the left of your anger focus) point at your target and really *shout*:

> *Don't YOU, EVER, EVER, EVER*
> *Let ME catch YOU*
> *Cleaning THAT CAT'S TEETH*
> *With MY toothbrush*
> *AGAIN!*

It is best to learn and talk through the words first before really throwing out your anger with real venom. Otherwise you may be fumbling to remember the words rather than putting real weight behind your expression of anger. Often, after four or five attempts, you will feel a flushing throughout your body as your anger begins to free up a physiological 'rearrangement'! It is quite common to develop a croaky throat after the exercise. You may need to do it several times over two or three days. As anger comes up, so you must shed it. If you are concerned about disturbing the neighbours then you can let the neighbours know that you are going to make a brief noise.

In 1987 I was in St Petersburg (then Leningrad) and I was invited to a coaching session at the Vaganova Ballet School – which provides dancers for the Maly and Kirov ballet companies – by one of the professors of dance. At the end of an hour's class the Professor harshly criticized three of the dancers and reduced them to tears. When the dancers had gone I asked him why he had been so angry. He said he was angry because they hadn't danced well. I asked him again why he was *so* angry. He said: 'I've just told you – because they didn't do very well. You were here and I wanted them to do well.' I explained that they had done very well as far as I was concerned and I suggested that he had actually come in angry and needed somewhere to 'hang' it. He looked surprised. We had a discussion about anger and solutions for it and I recommended the 'cat's teeth' exercise. I demonstrated the cat's-teeth exercise in the long training room with mirrors on all four walls and it was a peculiar experience. He stood and watched.

Two days later I was due to meet him again. He came bounding across the ground towards us with a smile on his face. He then explained that he had demonstrated and subsequently instructed the whole class in the cat's-teeth exercise. Ten years later I was back in St Petersburg and was invited to the ballet. After an excellent performance of *Swan Lake* at the Maly Ballet, I was invited backstage to meet some of the staff. As I walked along the wide corridor at the back of the theatre there were groups of dancers who seemed to be smiling as I went past them. I could not see any obvious reason so I asked my friend and he said: 'they have been doing the cats'-teeth exercise and we told them that the man who first mentioned it is here tonight in the audience!' It's a small exercise, but it packs enough punch to raise a smile after ten years!

So the cat's teeth exercise, one of many anger tools, is an exercise which is straightforward and available to all. It is an ideal tool to offload anger that might otherwise stress someone enough to prevent effective body repair and allow illness to begin. The great value of this exercise is that it converts anger into the absurd. Thereafter, if an incident that might normally have made you angry occurs, you need only think of the exercise to dispel the anger and stop it getting the better of you. Children love to do the exercise! What a gift it may be to teach children how to deal safely with anger before they find a more destructive way of unleashing it.

Unexpressed grief

Having shed your anger in a safe, quick and portable way, the next load to remove is unexpressed grief. More often than not, inpatients with cancers I have found that grief arises from unexpressed feelings about the death of someone close (often their parents) perhaps many years ago. Unexpressed grief may have weighed on their mental –

and physical – system for years. People often feel acute remorse at not having said more to the deceased before death. 'I wish that I had said that before he/she died'. This sentiment needs to be off loaded, and I suggest the following exercise.

Bereavement letter

Choose someone whom you trust to help with this exercise. Write a letter to the person you wish you had said things to before they died. Write this letter as if they were still alive. Acknowledge all the good things that happened during the time that they were alive: things you shared; lessons learned; moments of magic and tender times. Do this in the present tense as if they were still alive. Of any 'bad' memories, you should write only of *your feelings*. You may be recalling something very grim but for this exercise what matters are your feelings about it, not issues of right or wrong. For example, you might choose to say: 'when you threw me across the room I felt miserable'. This is better than 'you were wrong to throw me across the room'. So write about all the good things and your feelings about the bad things as you see them. This exercise may take about half an hour. It may be a very tearful process but that is a measure of the value you will have from finishing it. You will then be armed with a piece of paper, which may have been very painful to write.

Now you are going to make use of your throat chakra again.

With your chosen friend I suggest that you stand and read out the letter with them in the room. Their only job is to be there while you read the letter. When you have finished they should hug you until you are 'complete'. You are left with the paper in your hand (and probably your handkerchief in the other!).

You have a choice of what to do next. One option may be to set fire to the letter from a candle and to allow the letter to burn in the fireplace or other safe place. You can then leave the candle to burn down in its own time. The burning candle could be seen as the 'postal service' sending your letter to those who you wish you had spoken to before they died. If you use a 'cathedral' candle you might have several days to wait before it has burned down!

This exercise can be performed to resolve grief for lovers, partners, relatives or children (and even for a foetus that has been terminated).

Sometimes people undergo radical change in their lives (maybe because of injury or shock) and those around them may need to grieve for the person they once knew: the 'earlier' version. Of course, when this exercise is done for a living recipient, a decision needs to be made: whether only to read the document or whether to commit the document to the post. There can be some dramatic results if such a document is posted!

Finding 'your sound'

One exercise can help enormously to express bottled up feelings. Stand facing a friend and ask him to sound a note, as if singing. You then sound back the note, acting as an echo. You mirror whatever your friend does. Try 'sounding' a number of different notes until you find one that you feel is *your* note. Gradually, over the course of a few minutes, you may well find a note that absolutely resonates with you.

I can remember the first time that I did this exercise with a hard-nosed businessman. He was beginning to think that the exercise was futile. However, I could sense that he was almost deliberately fluctuating each side of a note that seemed to be closer to his resonant frequency – as if he was afraid of what might happen if he touched 'his' note. When he did sound the note he immediately broke down in tears, and he continued to cry for the next five minutes. Some months later he described this as having been a major turning point in his life. Many people start laughing – and keep going!

'Contacting the soul' through the eyes

Your innermost feelings may be close to your 'soul'. If eyes really are the windows of the soul then it may be helpful to reach your soul – or indeed let someone else reach it – through your eyes. This can be a very powerful exercise.

Sit facing somebody so that your knees are touching, holding hands. You then hold the person's gaze for perhaps two minutes. You will tend to deflect your eyes from one of their eyes to the other. Many things may happen. You may perceive changes in the age of their face. Some people have extraordinary and deep experiences during this process. Some people find it difficult. It is an easy exercise to describe, but can be difficult to perform. The rewards can be great.

This exercise can lead to a 'realization' of such importance that it accelerates the healing process. I remember doing this exercise with a patient who gained so much from it that the 'penny dropped', and no further action was needed to launch them on the road to recovery. Two years later she was completely well and regarded that one exercise as the turning point.

Exploring of the hands

Again you need a partner. Close your eyes and 'explore' your partner's hand with your fingers – to see just how much you can learn about them from their hands alone. This is a perfectly safe exercise and even more remarkable when done with a complete stranger. With someone you know you may gain a great insight about him or her beyond anything you have had before. During this process you need to allow yourself to receive as much information about them as you can. To start with you may notice only the skin texture, moisture and structure of their fingers and so on, but towards the end of the exercise you may find that you are being much more intuitive about the information you receive from them.

After the exercise you can let your partner know what information you have gleaned. In this way you have acted as a 'mirror' for them. They can then go through the same process with your hand. They then act as your mirror. In this way a relatively simple exercise may give you significant insights which may be very helpful. The first time I did this exercise I learned from the lady who 'explored' my hand that she felt a combination of humour and a desperation to help others! She was moved to tears when I told her what I had gleaned from hers. Some weeks later she sent me a book thanking me for insights that she had found very helpful.

These exercises can free you to discover important feelings that have been suppressed and whose suppression may have contributed to the development of disease. Much energy is tied up in suppression – rather like trying to push down the lid on a saucepan of boiling water.

Visualization

We have already seen the possible effectiveness of visualization in the lemon-segment exercise. The ability to picture imaginary scenes vividly stimulates your imagination and helps the mind influence the body's recovery. There are a large number of books, tapes, CDs and even videos to help people perform visualization exercises. Normally a visualization exercise is a passive experience. You sit quietly and enter a guided process with clear, easy-to-follow instructions. In time you may become familiar with specific visualizations and go through the process without guidance. But be careful which visualizations you use. Visualizations of illness being attacked and destroyed by aggressive forces are a mistake; this simply puts yourself under attack.

Here is a visualization that I have found helpful for patients who are 'stuck' in illness:

Imagine that it is early morning and that you are walking through a forest in the hills along a pine needle-strewn path. The sun is shining through the trees and lighting the rocks across the valley opposite. As you enjoy the walk you can hear the rumble of a waterfall just around the next corner. You are becoming warm as the morning heat begins to rise with the climbing sun. You turn the corner and see that your path crosses below the waterfall so that you will be soaked if you continue. You decide to undress and to throw your clothes in your bag on to the path just the other side of the waterfall. As you undress you enjoy a feeling of freedom. You undress, place your clothes carefully in the small backpack you have with you and throw it to the path on the other side of the waterfall. You then walk into the tumbling chute of water and stand still, enjoying the refreshing and cleansing sensation of the water. The strong roar of the water is stimulating for you. You notice the sun turning the drops of water spray into as many fireworks. You savour the waterfall for a while longer before deciding to continue across to the path on the other side. Quickly you dry and put on your clothes again, before setting off once again along the path through the trees.

A short while further along the path you reach a wooden hut, like a mountain hut, on the side of the path. The door is open and your curiosity draws you to it. The smell of the wood fire lingers inside the hut. The sun is shining through one of the windows. You feel the rough texture of the wood as you open the door enough to walk inside. Except for a wooden table and some chairs the hut is empty. You are about to leave when you notice a box on the table with a piece of paper resting against it. You walk to the table and see that the paper has your name on it and suggests that you open the box as the contents are for you and that it is for you to take with you. You lift the lid on the box and find inside it something very special for you. You pick it up and reflect for a moment what an extraordinary blessing this is for you. You pause for a moment to thank the hut and then you leave, closing the door a little behind you. You resume your walk towards the next village. Just before you leave the forest, and when you can first hear the sounds of the village, you stop to sit on a rock on the side of the path and pause for a few minutes to reflect before joining the path to the village.

At this stage you can check the ground is firm beneath your feet and, in your own time, open your eyes to rejoin the room.

Often, after the sense of cleansing from the waterfall,

people find a wonderful clue for them in the box in the hut. There is much scope to 'debrief' people on their experiences during the exercise and such debriefings can be enormously helpful in guiding patients.

Meditation

We have already mentioned meditation as one of the strategies of success. In contrast to visualization, which is a guided process where the listener is actively steered along a path, meditation attempts to create a void in the head from which thought is excluded. Again, the shelves are full of books and tapes on how to meditate. In these there is sometimes a self-righteousness about the 'right way to meditate'. The only 'right way' is a way that works for you. It may take some trial and error to find such a way.

My personal preference is to take advantage of a normal rhythmic process in the body. For me, early meditation is best done sitting in a 'sensible' chair without arms, with my feet firmly on the floor. My back is supported. It is easiest if my eyes are closed and my hands resting gently on my thighs. Next I observe my breathing. Is it faster or slower, deeper or shallower than the breath before? I apply this checklist to each subsequent breath as if I had a clipboard in front of me and I was marking the characteristics of one breath in relation to the breath before. By focusing on this internal rhythmic process, my mind is 'internalized' into one of its own body processes.

When people first try this meditation they may feel, after the first few 'cycles', that they've mastered the technique. Their minds will begin to drift to other thoughts. This prevents the 'void' forming. So to begin with, it is useful to have somebody in the room to watch you and occasionally remind you to return to your breathing. Likewise, it may help to regard any external sound (a bird chirping, a car passing) as your 'coach' reminding you to return to the exercise. Easy as it is to describe, this exercise is hard to do. Like a sport it is more difficult at first than it is later. The benefits of meditation are enormous. At a basic level it allows the body to focus on its own repair rather than on the humdrum activities of everyday life.

Neurolinguistic programming (NLP)

NLP combines physical stimulation with verbal suggestion to produce a physical result. It demonstrates very clearly how the state of your morale can effect your bodily strength and contains a range of techniques, some of which may be useful in jogging patients out of a rut. For example, allowing them to *associate* a good feeling with a particular colour, word or sound, a patient can be given the means to experience good feelings when they would not normally be able to. You can create triggers of many kinds to recall pleasant, useful and encouraging feelings and counteract feelings of vulnerability and depression. One of the most enjoyable series of courses that I have taken part in was created by Anthony Robbins (author of *Unlimited Power* and *Awaken the Giant Within*).

There are many workshops where the techniques of NLP are taught. NLP is sometimes extended to a process known as neuro-associative conditioning. The aim of these processes in the context of this book is to strengthen your ability to use your body to look after itself better.

Kinesiology

'Kinesiology' can be used to demonstrate or test effects of thoughts or substances on the body. This exercise shows how quickly the body can regain its power:

Ask somebody to stand with eyes closed and to extend their arm sideways. Ask them to keep it there, resisting you as you attempt to push the arm down to their side. Having obtained an indication of the strength required by you, allow them to lower the arm to their side. After a while, ask them to close their eyes and to remember a time when they felt really grim. Then ask them if they see this memory in black-and-white or in colour. If it is in black and white then it is probably an appropriate memory for this exercise. Ask them to put their arm out sideways and again attempt to push down while asking them to resist you. Often it will literally fall to their side.

You then ask them to lower that arm to their side, if it is not already there, and to shake both arms around for a bit before closing their eyes. Now ask them to lift their chin, stick out their chest and recall a time when they felt fantastic, confident and successful. You invite them to savour that feeling for a moment, remembering how it felt, who was there and so on. Then ask them to put out the arm once more and to try to resist your attempt to push it down. This time it is unlikely you will succeed in moving it at all!

This exercise demonstrates how powerful positive thought can be. Imagine how effective a positive thought process held for a while can be in creating a persistent 'healing' signal for the body.

Art therapy

For some people expressing their feelings by voice can be too difficult, but they may be able to express their feelings in paint or clay. While I was at the Bristol Cancer Help Centre, where there were excellent art therapists, there were two main art sessions during the course of the residential week. At the first session patients were invited to paint their illness as they saw it and felt it then. At the second session, later in the week, they were invited to paint an image as they subsequently felt.

The results were extraordinary. There are many ways of enjoying art as a form of therapy but it may appeal more to some people than others (just as with all the exercises mentioned). Once people had overcome the fear that they might be expected to paint 'well' they entered into the spirit of the exercise! For many it can be a very powerful exercise that can also double as a tool of exploration. It is hardly a major investment to buy some paints and paper to see if art helps to unlock an illness that has become entrenched.

If you really insist on that same daily commute!

Try taking a different way to and from work every day for two weeks. This move in itself may open the possibility of new encounters and perspectives.

Quick change from a depressed state!

Try to make the corners of your mouth go upwards without smiling!

A 'No' day

One characteristic of people who develop a malignancy is that they are often thought to be 'nice'. They are helpful to others and often seem to do things for others – 'always so helpful'.

Inside they may feel very different, but, sensitive to others, may never express annoyance or anger. They continue to oblige and find it very hard to say 'no'. This may be especially common in the 'giving' professions – teaching and nursing, for example.

I recommend that patients mark a day in their diaries on which they agree with themselves to decline every request made of them – even if it is as simple as 'pass the sugar'. By the end of the day they will have developed ways of rejecting requests *gently*. In doing so they will have regained their freedom of choice.

A 'Yes' day

It might be fun to review a pre-chosen day and to consider what might have happened if you had accepted all the invitations/requests made of you that day!

Chanting affirmation

In his several books, Wayne Dyer describes many exercises that can be used to confirm, consolidate and amplify a clear goal. He recommends one in particular. This is to chant 'aaaah' confidently *while visualizing your desired goal*. Hold the 'aaaah' until running out of air and then start again with the same focus and a strong sound. You can repeat this process for as long as you wish. It helps to achieve a moment of reinforced focus for a minimum of ten minutes to half an hour. Doing this every day has a reinforcing tendency. Again, the aim is to move *forwards* to the chosen goal rather than away from something you are trying to avoid.

Colour

A regular feature of cancer patients in the time soon after diagnosis is that they often wear 'subdued' clothing. Blacks and dark blues were regular choices at the Help Centre at the beginning of a residential course week. Towards the end of the week brighter colours were appearing!

I suggest that they people who are feeling 'down' try wearing bright colours.

I remember seeing two ladies in their seventies, both going through the cancer experience, who were afraid of ridicule from their families. When I suggested that they might like to explore wearing brightly coloured clothes, one lady in particular said that her daughter would probably criticize her. She was adamant that she could not wear bright colours. I suggested that on their way home she could stop at a smart lingerie shop and buy herself some brightly coloured silk underwear. She could then stand right next to her intimidating daughter knowing that the daughter was unaware of her mother's sudden outburst of colour! She could feel that she was defying her daughter – even in some way defeating her – and all this in an atmosphere of good humour. Gradually she might develop the courage to wear more colourful outer clothing. This seemed to strike a note with her and her whole demeanour changed.

Sound of music

Just as visual change can be valuable, so too can a change of music or of the voices of those you choose to be with. If you want to feel 'down' then choose the company of people who depress your spirits, play slow, minor key music, wear dark clothes, live in a dark house and stick to routines.

If you seek change, then wear bright clothes with colour, listen to uplifting music, let light into the house (or go on a sunny holiday), change your routines and mix with people whose company stimulates you. There are all sorts of musical exercises to help. Laughter workshops, also, help people regain a light-heartedness that they may not have felt for some time.

The six-month diary

I mentioned this earlier as a tool to help guide people to discover what really matters for them as they make a future mission.

Picture yourself wherever you would most like to be in six months time. Write a review of the intervening six months as if they have turned out in the best possible way for you.

There are some rules:

- *Be unreasonable.* If you include only what you believe to be possible you are neither stretching your boundaries nor being true to your ambitions.

- *Make sure there are no 'steps' to an outcome.* A 'step' is a hurdle. An example of this is '(a) must happen before (b) can'. That implies that you can perceive only one way of reaching (b). Don't restrict yourself. Go direct to (b) and leave your options open on how to get there.

• *Do not live anyone else's life for them.* Don't fall back to organizing other's lives. For this exercise do not drag them into your plans either. In a 'relationship' scenario (home, friends or work), if you do not know what to do then I suggest you include something along the lines of, 'by . . . month X and I had reached the perfect relationship for us, and were both very happy with it'.

• *Make the six months enjoyable.* This is the most commonly forgotten part. Why make it all struggle and no fun?

Stand up and read your diary out aloud to someone else. Be proud of it! You made it! You will notice bits that seem to ring true for you and your observer will hear your intonation and emphasis. This may provide a clue to what particularly drives you or excites you. Verbalizing it helps to 'activate' it for you and by reading it out aloud to someone else you create an ally to help you reach your goals.

Address solutions, not problems

I remember one lady at the Bristol Cancer Help Centre who was on a week's course, but who had a 'result' from just one comment on the morning of her first day.

She was airing her unfortunate (as she saw it) life and commented on how bad things were in her marriage and work. I told her that it seemed as if it would be a relief for her to die. She asked me angrily: 'Why do you think that?'

I told her that it appeared that she would like to end her marriage and leave her job because both seemed to be so bad. She was visibly taken aback and said: 'they're not *that* bad, but I need to air it all the time.'

I asked: 'Is any of your life worthwhile?'

She said: 'Yes, of course.'

I suggested: 'Why not live and talk about the life you ARE having and wish to have, not the life you are 'not' having and do not enjoy?'

So, if you have difficulty in fixing on a plan, address the challenges in your life as *questions* on how to solve them. For example, what would it take to achieve a result? How would it become enjoyable again? These are 'empowering' questions, and are far more likely to reach a result than dwelling on your disadvantages.

How others can help – a 'round robin'

If you are a supporter or partner of someone who is seriously ill there is another very powerful gift you can give them.

Contact as many of their friends as you can and ask them to write down the two or three things they like best about the person you wish to help. Have them put their name on the piece of paper. Collect all their comment papers and take or send these to the person you are caring for. Let that person read them out aloud. If they cannot read then the contributors could put their comments on tape. The effect is often enormous.

*

These are just a handful of the available exercises, each one of them a potential turning point. Tom Lehrer once alluded to a friend of his who said that 'life was like a sewer' because 'you only got out of it what you put into it'! Treat the exercises in the same way – if you want a result put yourself right into it. If you only half attempt something you can expect only half a result.

Astrology?

I have known patients who found that 'having their own chart done' helped lift the mirror for them at a time when they could see no solutions. Relatively cheaply, a full 'personality profile' can be done and some 'transits' for the year ahead, for example. Sensibly used, this becomes an idea generator and a number of patients have found it to provide 'explanations' for them. Equinox of Covent Garden are one company providing this service. They offer another product, 'Astro*Carto*Graphy', with which they help to pinpoint geographic locations which are strong for that individual, whether good or bad. For a small outlay it may be helpful.

If things seem irreversible

Sometimes the situation can look very bleak indeed. For patient, family and friends, despair can destroy all hope of a good outcome. In that situation a valuable exercise for both the patient and his immediate circle is for each person to 'clear their stuff'. That means sitting with the sick person, preferably making body contact, and stating what was particularly enjoyable about knowing them. This does not need to be a huge list, but just a few points. If talking is too hard, silent contact with the intention of transferring feeling may help.

These exchanges, like the 'round robin' letter described above, can make a great difference to the patient's state. In addition, by having this exchange beforehand, the grief of not having spoken freely that often afflicts the bereaved is avoided if the sick person should die. Should the discussion lead to the recovery of the patient, the added bonus is that the relationship between them is much more open!

Moss Reports

Dr Ralph Moss has produced an excellent series of 'reports' for a wide range of cancers. The reports contain information on specific cancers and information on what has been tried in mainstream medicine with evidence 'for' and 'against', as well as other unorthodox solutions with evidence 'for' and 'against'. As a means of equipping patients for meetings with doctors and others and in helping them to understand the basis of any treatments offered, I regard these reports as extremely helpful.

Fenzian Treatment

There are many forms of medical treatment used for cancers. One which I have found highly effective in treating patients after surgery is the Fenzian electrical impulse treatment. Healing rates after surgery were much faster and uncomfortable consequences of radiotherapy and chemotherapy were frequently reduced. It was a great contribution to rehabilitation.

Chapter 6
Case Studies

Cancers can affect all sorts of people in all occupations and of any age, and in this chapter I shall explore how different people have faced their illness and what might be learned from their stories. What is most important to recognize is that although the causes of cancer are often complex, there are often certain 'triggers' or pressures in a patient's life that have loaded their immune system for too long.

Sometimes the site of a cancer may help in the search for underlying unresolved pressures or worries. For example, a kidney problem might indicate strong fear; breast cancer a difficulty with 'nurturing' relationships; backs with money worries and intestines with a sense of insurmountable loads.

Often, simply talking with someone about life leading up to the illness can help highlight what it is in the patient's life that has triggered that illness.

In the examples below, certain themes recur. There are people who give more than they receive, people who do not want to upset others and people who feel impotent in the face of 'establishment'.

It may be a strange thing to do to dwell on the cause of the cancer, but the whole process can act as a valuable catalyst both in self-understanding and further treatment. The discovery of a trigger for the cancer can result in patients gaining a sense of 'meaning' from the illness. Greater understanding can also have very practical benefits in helping the patient to change habits that may have contributed to the illness in the first place.

Jane

Jane was an adventurer. She arranged unusual holidays in a wide range of countries for groups of enthusiasts. Nothing was more enjoyable for her than to be guiding her group around a route that she had agreed and planned with them months earlier. She had begun to make this a way of life and it had helped to fill the gaps when her husband was away on business. He was an ex-military man working as a merchant banker.

Jane came for help when she had already been operated on for intestinal cancer that had spread to her liver. When I spoke of the triggers, she went very quiet and said that her husband's retirement meant that he was at home all the time. He also felt emasculated by no longer working in the 'City' and expected her to be a personal assistant to him. Jane was a 'giver' and thought it was the strain of always trying to please him, as a 'corporate wife' that had led to her illness. Her husband chose not to consider any 'non-medical' approaches and I could only help Jane directly.

She became very sad that he could see no point in broadening the approaches but said it had always been that way. He would throw any amount of money at 'proper' treatment 'because he was her husband' but could not see her as an individual with her own wishes and needs. Thanks to her exploring her pain and trying to understand the causes of it, she reached a stage where she was very much at peace with herself. She wanted to talk about death because she was 'ready' for it. She died peacefully and without any more pain.

I understood that Jane was a wild, vivacious lady when she became married and loved having children, but had increasing difficulties, losing her identity to 'corporate wifedom'. Her wild streak was constrained by having to conform and the expression of her own wishes and identity took second place.

There is often a great fear of two people discussing changing needs and feelings. All too often they feel it is wrong not to feel the way they did when they first became a partnership. Different people move at different speeds and in different directions. The dynamics of 'modern' life make it much harder for two people to remain on a relatively synchronized path and the strains of trying to force the paths to go together can be enormous.

Simon

Simon was playing professionally as a musician at concerts when he heard that he had to pay more than a million pounds to Lloyd's of London insurance company 'because of their incompetence and corruption'. His entire possessions amounted to £156,000 but he tried to press on with his work to find a way of paying what they demanded of him. This went on for two years as he sold his house and all his other assets, moving with his wife (who needed a hip replacement) to a caravan that he parked on a friend's farm. He offered what help he could on the farm to try to repay the farmer for allowing him to be there. Lloyd's continued to hound him for money throughout the following winter.

He felt he was feeling the cold more than he normally would have. He began to lose weight and suddenly found that he was passing blood when he emptied his bladder. The following day he came to me and I guided him through his hospital investigations as an emergency that afternoon. He was found to have a cancer in one of his kidneys and he had it removed. When I saw him after he left hospital he told me that he had returned home (to his caravan) to a pile of further demands for money from Lloyd's. He could not pay them.

I enlisted the help of another patient who was a lawyer to help build his support team. The advice he was given was to declare bankruptcy and his debt chapter would finally close. He was very reluctant to do so as he was worried that if he could not pay, someone else might have to make up for him and he would be letting down others. It became clear that he had little option but to admit in a means test that he could not pay any more. After completing all the paperwork he began to put on weight and was in excellent shape when I saw him again four years later.

I have frequently seen people developing serious illnesses at times when the pressure of financial worries has been too great. A combination of sharing the worries he had and also enlisting the help of professional advice eased the load on his mind and gave his body a chance. As is frequently the case, for those who recover, he found himself subsequently choosing to help others!

Gareth

I first met Gareth when he came to me with stomach trouble. He was an estate agent with a great enthusiasm for helping people find the right house, working with his accountant brother in the business that their father had left to them when he had died three years earlier. Gareth was delightful and gentle; clients liked him enormously and he frequently found himself helping people because it was in his nature. I even remember him driving a client to Cambridge from Bristol because they had a problem with their car and the trains would have been too slow to carry them there in time! It was just his nature to help people. His brother was not the same and, although Gareth was the one whose approach brought in the clients, his brother increasingly tried to 'expand the business'. His brother drove Gareth hard, criticizing his apparently 'time-wasting' approach when he was talking with people. The difference between them grew. Gareth felt terrible because on the one hand he wanted to fulfil his brother's demands and, on the other, he wanted to be his old helpful self. When I felt his stomach I could feel a lump. Rapid investigation led to the timely removal of a malignant growth in his colon. He has been well ever since, but he realized that he needed to change his work pattern.

Had he returned to his previous job he would, in my view, have had 'recurrences'. One driving force for the original problem would still have been unaltered. Instead, he set up shop on his own and created a happy business where he regained his old persona and was doing well at the time of writing. Because of his friendly ways he had steady 'support' from the community he created around him.

Businesses – and especially family businesses – can cause undue strain to an individual. Sometimes you need to forsake tradition and change if you are going to avoid a recurrence.

Jonathan

Jonathan first visited me after collapsing on the pavement outside the building in the City where he had worked for thirty-seven years. It was 7.45 in the morning and many people, including some working in his own department, walked past him, assuming that he was a drunk! Finally, a wonderful lady who had worked in his building for many years helped him to his feet and into work. He broke down and said that he had not been feeling well for some time. It seems that he had been suffering at work for some time because of homophobic and professionally libellous comments about him spread by malicious colleagues. The cancer he had was untreatable and had already spread to his spine. The weakness from this disease had led to his collapse in the street.

I looked after him in the few months which remained before he died and he declared many times that he felt that the illness had arisen as a result of the nastiness which came from colleagues. He lived alone so he also had less chance of sharing his troubles. He was also insistent that he did not want to become a 'problem' to others if he should become incapacitated, and he took an overdose.

Perhaps Jonathan would have done better if he had felt able to express his feelings earlier amongst a group of friends or with a professional or clergyman. I think the battering that he felt he had had at the hands of his colleagues had driven him into a corner. In the loneliness that followed, the problems brewed inside him. His illness created a new forum in which he could talk about his difficulties, but by then he had no energy left to start a new life. Also, his absolute dedication to his job took place at the expense of any hobbies. He had no hobbies with which to dilute the work situation or hobbyists to share his predicament.

David

David worked in a well-known merchant bank. He had handled many clients and was under the usual pressure to pull money into the bank. However, the highest 'growth area' of clients available to the bank were those bringing funds from crime; in particular drug dealing and people smuggling from Eastern Europe. The Financial Authorities declare rigid rules to ensure that banks identify the origin of the funds that are to be kept in the bank accounts but a conflict of interests arose when some well-suited visitors asked to open an account. They wanted to deposit $50m in the bank 'as a first instalment'. They told David that they knew about the rules but understood from a friend of the chairman that a cash payment of around 2 per cent normally sorted the 'administrative difficulties' of those rules!

He chose to seek advice from senior staff and was told that they could not officially sanction him accepting money like this but that 'all the banks were doing it'. They told him that the money 'would only be taken elsewhere' if they did not accept it! He was put under great pressure to bend the rules in the bank's interest, providing he was not seen to be doing it. He was a classic 'fall guy'. As a grandfather, he was very anxious to pay for the education of his two grandchildren and to keep his job until retirement. When he retired he became ill with a tongue cancer and had major surgery to remove the tumour.

Unaware of his job situation, when I first spoke with him after the cancer (he was having to re-learn how to do this after losing much of his tongue), I asked if he had ever felt the need to express something but felt unable to do so. He asked why I asked and I told him that the problem he had had was at the level of the throat 'chakra' and this level was sometimes associated with difficulties in expression. He put his head in his hands and spoke of the secret burden he had found himself to be under for so many years. He had been afraid to speak to anyone about the work problems and had 'bottled it up'. To 'confess' seemed to help enormously. Most of the difficulty appeared to hang on the suppression of rage at the bank and at how he had felt the need to do many things he would rather not have done to ensure the security of his job and income for his grandchildren. He found the cat's-teeth exercise enormously helpful and has had a good past five years in which he has used his experience to help others.

It must have been very tough for David to find himself caught in a 'Firm' like his merchant bank. He had become a pawn of the bank where his vulnerability on producing adequate 'performance' controlled every waking hour. As his outgoings grew with his grandchildren's education he found that the organization that he had been taught so to respect was a sham. Not only were they happy to take on corrupt clients, but they were happy to use non-Board employees to act as fall guys. Retiring freed him from them. 'Confessing' helped to unload the burden for him, allowing his body to heal again. He had great abilities and might well have been able to resign at the first flicker of corruption, but he did not feel confident of creating a new life so close to retirement. He was lucky that his 'problem' arose at a time when his life had to change on that retirement! He could offload the worries and start a more harmonious existence.

Debbie

Debbie was forty-five when she first visited me, having just had a mastectomy for breast cancer. She was in a programme of chemotherapy and had finished her course of radiotherapy. Her hair had fallen out and her self-esteem was at rock bottom. Although she had followed the medical recommendations, her primary worry was that nobody had been able to discuss what might have led to the cancer forming in the first place. She was the wife of a hard-working businessman and had maintained the role of a 'corporate wife' for many years. It turned out that she had also experienced a difficult relationship with her own mother, who seemed to have found children difficult to handle within her life as a 'corporate wife'. When she had her own children she had tried to mother them 'properly' and felt she might almost have smothered them. They left home when she was forty and she found herself suddenly alone, wondering what she was going to do with her life. She felt her son and daughter ought now to be around for her. She felt abandoned and could find solace from neither her mother nor her children. Not only had she not felt 'nurtured' by her own mother but she felt rejected by the 'children' she had nurtured and to whom she had dedicated a number of her years.

It turned out that she had made her children a distracting 'project' (meaning she could put off decisions about her own life). She had also decided to 'over-mother' her children to spite her own mother – she would 'show her how it should have been done!' Ultimately, they were fed up with being swamped by their mother flooding them with presents, clothes and interference paid for by 'Dad'. Debbie felt rejected. We therefore discussed how she could choose and begin a life that stimulated her. We worked out how to put her in a situation where others valued her for who she was and what she could do. It was only with such changes that she began to feel better. She became the manager of a local hotel and created a family atmosphere where she felt very much valued.

To say that breast cancers are of a 'nurturing' organ might seem trite, but it seems quite common, in my experience, for women with breast cancers to have unresolved issues. These usually relate either to what they perceive to be a poor relationship with their mothers or with their children, especially when their children leave home and no longer need 'nurturing' as they did before. By resolving these issues some valuable energy becomes available to help heal them. It would seem to be less valuable only to treat them as medical cases and to ignore possible precipitating (and soluble) issues.

Sam

I was asked to see Sam when he was eight years old. He was in hospital, having developed a cancer for the second time. Curiously, the new cancer was of a very different type and was regarded as a completely new illness.

Sam was in bed playing computer games. His father was egging him on to score maximum points. The father seemed to be so absorbed in instructing Sam that he ignored me coming in and saying hello. Eventually, Sam did well enough at his game. I spoke with them for a while and discovered that Sam had a 'golden' sister who was ten years old, a 'high-achiever' to whom excellence in bookwork and sport seemed to come naturally. I had some simple treatment equipment that I believed might help Sam and showed him how to use it. I said I would call back. Three days later I returned and found Sam's mother there. The equipment had not been used and I asked why. Sam's mother told me that her husband had totally researched all the chemotherapy programmes for Sam and distrusted anything else. I told Sam and his father that I would take away the equipment as they were not using it but that I would bring it back immediately if they told me they wanted it.

Sam's family was heavily involved in their community and I sensed very strongly that Dad wanted Sam to equal, or exceed, his sister's abilities. I told the mother that I was worried about undue pressure on Sam. His mother broke down and told me that Sam's father had pushed him from the beginning and that he 'drove by criticism'. Sam could only attract the full attention of both parents from his sister when he was ill. I suggested that if his father let him off the hook of achievement and stopped driving him then he might improve quite quickly. She said she '*knew* it was the problem'. I told her that Sam might be using the illness in two ways: first, to have the attention that he felt he could not otherwise earn and second, that he might fear never achieving his father's standards; it would be easier to die rather than let him down. In spite of attempts to encourage a different approach to Sam's illness, his mother dared not raise it with the father. The fear of tackling him made me more convinced of how great the pressure had been. Sam did not 'respond' to his treatment in hospital and died four months later.

Imagine how it might have been had Sam's father told him that he loved his son anyway, regardless of whether he 'succeeded' at school or not. He could have taken the immense pressure to 'achieve' off his son and Sam might have felt able to face life more strongly. It is just possible that he would not have needed the illness to gain the affection he so badly wanted.

Chapter 7
Maintaining
the Momentum

We sometimes 'chase up' patients who we have not heard from for a while to see how they are doing. This is not so much to check on their illness (preferably their past illness) as to see how they are doing in their life mission. Normally this is only a short call but it is invariably well received. You could easily call a couple of friends to see how they are doing – just put a note on your calendar to do it. Recently, I called one patient who had been under huge stress running his own business, earning nothing and becoming increasingly ill. We had spoken at length about change but he had not felt able to at that time. Two years later, I had only his mobile phone number. When he answered he sounded very cheerful and I asked how things were. He told me that he had sold the business, teamed up with a previous work colleague and was sailing in the Mediterranean. He was sitting on a sailing yacht (a long-held dream of his) as I called! He believed that by fulfilling a long felt wish his illness had left him alone.

By creating these 'virtual' support communities we can generate more enjoyable lives. It is possible that community support will give us good health as well. We become each other's teachers and mirrors, so that when we are 'up' we can support those who are not. When we need support, they might just be there to help us!

I hope something in the book has helped you. Good luck, wherever you are on your path.

Additional Information

Anthony Robbins:
www.anthonyrobbins.com

Joan Borysenko and Miroslav Borysenko:
The Power of the Mind to Heal: Renewing Body, Mind and Spirit, Hay House, Inc., 1994

Ralph Moss:
www.ralphmoss.com
www.cancerdecisions.com

Equinox:
www.astrology.co.uk

Wayne Dyer:
www.drwaynedyer.com

Ute Brookman:
Argyle Herbs Direct, Severidges Farm, Waterrow, Taunton, Somerset TA4 2BH

Fenzian Treatment System:
www.fenzian.com

Index